MAGNETICALLY ASSISTED HEMODIALYSIS: A NEW STRATEGY FOR THE TREATMENT OF END STAGE RENAL DISEASE

MAGNETICALLY ASSISTED HEMODIALYSIS: A NEW STRATEGY FOR THE TREATMENT OF END STAGE RENAL DISEASE

D. STAMOPOULOS

D. BENAKI
P. BOUZIOTIS
C. KOTSOVASSILIS
AND

P.N. ZIROGIANNIS

Nova Science Publishers, Inc.
New York

For permission to use material from this book please contact us:
Telephone 631-231-7269; Fax 631-231-8175
Web Site: http://www.novapublishers.com

NOTICE TO THE READER

Library of Congress Cataloging-in-Publication Data
Available Upon Request
ISBN 978-1-60456-681-9

Published by Nova Science Publishers, Inc. ✜ New York

To my father Nikolaos
my mother Anna
my sister Maria
D. Stamopoulos

Contents

About the Authors

D. Stamopoulos
Author to whom any correspondence should be addressed
Tel.:+302106503330; *E-mail address:*densta@ims.demokritos.gr
Institute of Materials Science, NCSR "Demokritos", 153-10, Aghia Paraskevi, Athens, Greece

D. Benaki
Institute of Biology, NCSR "Demokritos", 153-10, Aghia Paraskevi, Athens, Greece

P. Bouziotis
Institute of Radioisotopes-Radiodiagnostic Products, NCSR "Demokritos", 153-10, Aghia Paraskevi, Athens, Greece

C. Kotsovassilis
Department of Clinical Biochemistry, General Hospital "G. Gennimatas", National Health System, 115-27, Athens, Greece

P.N. Zirogiannis
Department of Nephrology, General Hospital "G. Gennimatas", National Health System, 115-27, Athens, Greece

D. Stamopoulos, the primary author of the present book, would like to warmly thank his coauthors for the valuable help that they provided during the experimental work and for the constitutive comments that they provided while reviewing the manuscript

Preface

"Of all writings I love only that which is written with blood"
Of Reading and Writing
Thus spoke Zarathustra
F. Nietzsche

Biocompatible Ferromagnetic Nanoparticles (FNs) can be considered as objects of zero dimensions that owing to their extremely small size and intense magnetism are free to circulate in the human vascular network and eventually be focused at a specific area of interest under the application of an external magnetic field. Currently, FNs motivate many biotechnological/biomedical applications at a diagnostic level, as magnetic contrast agents for Magnetic Resonance Imaging, or even at a therapeutic stage, as carriers of radioisotopes and/or chemotherapeutic drugs for their targeted delivery to tumor tissues.

In the present book we introduce the utilization of FNs in the concept of Magnetically Assisted Hemodialysis (MAHD) for the treatment of End Stage Renal Disease (ESRD). ESRD patients have to be subjected to permanent Hemodialysis (HD) therapy having a typical schedule of three 4-hour sessions per week. The proposed strategy of MAHD aims to become a more efficient development of conventional HD. The core of the idea is the production of Ferromagnetic Nanoparticles-Targeted Binding Substance Conjugates (FN-TBS Cs) constructed of biocompatible FNs and a specifically designed TBS. The TBS part is used for increasing the biocompatibility of the FNs host carriers and should have high affinity and binding capacity for the specific Target Toxic Substance (TTS) that should be removed from the patient. For these demands to be fulfilled, antibodies or even specific proteins could serve as the TBS part of the desired FN-TBS Cs. The FN-TBS Cs should be administered to the patient timely prior to the MAHD session so that, owing to their free circulation in the vascular network, they will be able to collect the desired TTSs through their adsorption onto the TBS part of the Cs. However, long residence times of the FN-TBS Cs in the blood stream cannot be used so that noticeable triggering of the reticuloendothelial system to be avoided. As a result, the binding dynamics of the FN-TBS Cs with candidate TTSs are of major importance. Eventually, the complex FN-TBS-TTS can be selectively removed during the MAHD session by means of a "magnetic dialyser", that is a magnetic field device installed at the dialysis machine in series to the conventional dialyser.

The advantages of MAHD over conventional HD are discussed in detail among issues of practical importance. Some of the main advantages are the following: (i) increased rate of toxin removal, (ii) selective targeting of specific TTSs and prevention by the respective disorders during early stages, (iii) decreased duration of each dialysis session, and (iv) adjustment of the blood flow rate to relatively lower values. Apart from these primary benefits related to the comfort and overall health status of the patient, enormous financial benefits will also evolve for National Health Budgets since the proposed MAHD strategy requires small investments and only modest modification of existing dialysis machines.

We review results obtained by using Fe_3O_4 and Bovine Serum Albumin (BSA) as the FNs and the TBS constituents, respectively. By means of X-ray diffraction, Atomic Force Microscopy, Circular Dichroism spectropolarimetry, UV-VIS spectrophotometry, and SQUID magnetometry we have studied in great detail the structural/morphological and magnetic properties of the formed Fe_3O_4-BSA Cs. Specifically, by means of SQUID magnetometry we have evaluated the magnetic retraction efficiency of the produced Fe_3O_4-BSA Cs that is a key property for the realization of MAHD. Most importantly, by employing Circular Dichroism spectropolarimetry, UV-VIS spectrophotometry, Nuclear Magnetic Resonance, Fluorescence Polarization Immunoassay and Turbidimetry Immunoassay we have evaluated the toxin binding affinity and capacity of both bare Fe_3O_4 FNs and Fe_3O_4-BSA Cs by performing *in vitro* experiments on specific TTSs. Homocysteine, p-Cresol and β2-microglobulin have been investigated in great detail. Our investigations mainly refer to experiments that are performed in the laboratory. However, we have also performed mock-dialysis experiments by means of standard dialysers and dialysis machines that are used in HD practice. MAHD mock-dialysis experiments are presented for the evaluation of the magnetic retraction efficiency of the prepared Fe_3O_4-BSA Cs. Also we evaluated the removal efficiency of homocysteine by performing MAHD mock-dialysis experiments in comparison to conventional HD mock-dialysis ones. In the MAHD mock-dialysis experiments the "magnetic dialyser" was implemented by an array of permanent magnets placed along the extracorporeal blood circulation line. The obtained results prove the *in vitro* successful applicability of the proposed MAHD method.

We are grateful to the staff of the Dialysis Unit in the General Hospital "G. Gennimatas" for the hospitality. Especially, we are grateful to Nurses D. Michalopoulos and V. Galani for the important assistance they provided during the mock-dialysis experiments. We warmly thank the staff of the Dialysis Unit "Filoxenia" and especially Nephrologist K. Papadopoulos for assistance and enlightening discussions. Physician V. Dalamagas, Nephrologist Dr. A. Lagouranis, Physicist Dr. E. Manios and Electronic Engineer V. Vlessidis are warmly acknowledged for enlightening discussions and useful assistance that promoted the present work. Finally we wish to thank NOVA Science Publishers for offering us the opportunity to rapidly communicate to the readership the newly emerged MAHD concept.

We hope that the utilization of MAHD into clinical practice will become a reality so that long-term-HD patients will benefit from all the advantages discussed here, and from many more that will probably evolve after intense *in vivo* applications are completed.

D. Stamopoulos
December 2007
Institute of Materials Science
NCSR, "Demokritos"
Athens, Greece

Abbreviations

AFM	Atomic Force Microscopy
AGEPs	Advanced Glycation End Products
β2-m	β2-microglobulin
BSA	Bovine Serum Albumin
CD	Circular Dichroism
CKD	Chronic Kidney Disease
CVD	Cardiovascular Disease
Cys	Cysteine
DM	Diabetes Mellitus
DOQI	Dialysis Outcomes Quality Initiative
EMAHD	Extracorporeal MAHD
ESRD	End Stage Renal Disease
fHcy	free Hcy
fpC	free pC
FPIA	Fluorescence Polarization Immunoassay
FNs	Ferromagnetic Nanoparticles
FN-TBS Cs	Ferromagnetic Nanoparticle-Targeted Binding Substance Conjugates
GFR	Glomerular Filtration Rate
HC	Hypercholesterolemia
Hcy	Homocysteine
HD	Hemodialysis
HDP	HD Product
HSA	Human Serum Albumin
HT	Hypertension
MAHD	Magnetically Assisted Hemodialysis
MDRD	Modification-of-Diet-in-Renal-Disease
MS	Metabolic Syndrome
MTBS	Multi Targeted Binding Substance
MW	Molecular Weight
NMR	Nuclear Magnetic Resonance
pC	p-Cresol
RRF	Residual Renal Function
SQUID	Superconducting Quantum Interference Device
TBS	Target Binding Substance
tHcy	total Hcy
TIA	Turbidimetry Immunoassay
tpC	total pC
TTS	Target Toxic Substance
UV-VIS	Ultraviolet-Visible
URR	Urea Reduction Ratio
XRD	X-ray Diffraction

Chapter 1

Introduction

Hemodialysis (HD) has become a mature therapy owing to remarkable technical innovations related to sensor devices that drive automatically-controlled safety systems, to improvements on the biocompatibility of the disposable materials used in the extracorporeal circuit, and to utilization of effective medication. All these factors have enabled the significant reduction of possible side effects. However, these significant improvements cannot eliminate all the complications that accompany HD, so that many side effects still relate to this renal replacement modality.

The most fundamental drawback of HD possibly relates to its *intermitted* nature which is clearly unphysiologic. [1, 2] Currently, an international practice has been established which is scheduled at three 4-hour sessions per week. It is generally believed that such a schedule delivers an adequate dose of HD to the patient. However, it is obvious that this *intermittent* process cannot sustain adequately the *continuous* biological activities occurring in human body, ultimately resulting in suboptimal outcome when referring to both morbidity and mortality. The proposition of a more *physiological* HD therapy that is performed for longer duration on a daily basis has been introduced lately. [2–7] Ideally, increasing both the duration and the frequency of HD will allow delivering of significantly higher dialysis doses of less intermittent nature to the patient, thus improving his/her overall health status. However, such a schedule obviously downgrades both patient's comfort and quality-of-life. The significant inconvenience related to more frequent and long-duration HD could be overcome by novel artificial renal devices that aim to be both implantable/wearable and *continuously* functioning. [8–10] Such devices are currently designed and evaluated in *in vitro* experiments.

A second fundamental drawback of HD relates to its inefficiency to replace the complex metabolic, endocrine and immunological processes of the natural kidney. To sufficiently replace these lost functions, experimental efforts have been focused on the engineering of a *bioartificial* kidney that is based on the utilization of an extra membrane consisting of renal tubule cells. [10–16] This tissue-engineered membrane is placed in the extracorporeal circuit and is activated during HD. Humes and colleagues have performed *in vivo* applications using uremic dogs and confirmed that metabolic activity took place in the layer of renal tubular cells. [13] Late on, the first clinical applications were reported by the same group on acute-renal-failure patients. [16, 17]

The two drawbacks discussed above are currently studied at an experimental stage mainly in *in vitro* experiments and, in less extent, in *in vivo* applications in uremic animals. Their efficiency has been limitedly evaluated for the treatment of acute-renal-failure and multiple-organ-failure patients. However, owing to the interdisciplinary character of this highly sophisticated project, clinical trials on long-term-HD patients are still missing.

A third important drawback of HD relates to the incomplete removal of specific toxins by both the low- and high-flux dialysers that are currently used in this renal replacement modality. For instance, many low and middle molecular-weight (MW) toxins that have high affinity for blood-serum proteins are not removed efficiently by conventional dialysers. [18–22] The accumulation of these toxins in blood is associated with specific disorders. For instance, hyperhomocysteinemia [23–27] and amyloidosis [28–30] are two disorders that currently cannot be treated adequately, motivating serious health complications mainly related to cardiovascular disease (CVD). To overcome this inefficiency, sophisticated dialysers are currently manufactured that aim to remove target toxins of specific MW. [31–33] The membranes of these dialysers have narrow pore-size distribution focused around a desired value that is accurately controlled at the nanometer level. It is believed that these nanostructured membranes can efficiently remove these target toxins.

This third important drawback of HD has attracted our efforts. Very recently we introduced the concept of Magnetically Assisted Hemodialysis (MAHD) [see Refs. [34–37] and http://nanotechweb.org/cws/article/lab/32024] that can be employed for the selective and efficient removal of toxins that, although of high biological importance, they cannot be handled by current dialysers. MAHD is based on the utilization of Ferromagnetic Nanoparticles (FNs) in conventional HD. Before we refer to our work let us make a brief review on current biotechnological issues that are based on the utilization of FNs. Nowadays, FNs have been extensively studied in Materials Science due to their unique properties. As their name manifests, regarding their size these particles are crystallites that have extremely small dimensions in the range of nanometers. Owing to their noticeable magnetic susceptibility, FNs can be easily manipulated under the application of an external magnetic field. In addition, based on standard chemical methods not only their dimensions but also their shape can be controlled at will, ranging from nanometers to micrometers and from spherical to needle-like, respectively. Such FNs have been studied extensively in basic-research topics of Materials Science, [38–40] as efficient candidates for magnetic recording media, as constituents of magnetic-field-sensor devices, [41, 42] and also in biomedical applications. [43–57] During the recent decade it was recognized that FNs have a great potential for biomedical applications owing to their following specific characteristics: (i) Their small size enables not only their free circulation through the vascular network but also their intracellular delivery. (ii) Their biocompatibility is guarantied once the appropriate material is chosen. For instance, in reasonable amounts iron oxides (Fe_2O_3, Fe_3O_4) are by far the most well studied biocompatible FNs that interfere only weakly with the immune system. (iii) Their magnetic susceptibility enable their manipulation through the vascular network and eventually their focusing at a specific body regime by means of an external magnetic field. (iv) The tailoring of their hysteretic magnetic properties enable the control of the amount of heat that they can release to the surrounding tissue environment during successive magnetization loops under the application of an alternating magnetic field.

All these magnetic and morphological characteristics of FNs have been utilized in both *in vitro* and *in vivo* biomedical applications. As diagnostic tools FNs have been introduced successfully in the magnetic resonance imaging application for increasing the contrast between healthy and cancer tissues. [45, 46] Also, in therapeutic treatments they have been used in hyperthermia for the selective destruction of tumor tissues and for targeted delivery of drugs in chemo- and radiotherapy of cancer. [47–49] For a detailed presentation of these topics Refs. [50, 51, 54] could be consulted. Very recently, Fe_3O_4 FNs were introduced *in vitro* in an ultra sensitive detection technique for the early evaluation of slightly increased levels of C-reactive protein, a peptide that serves as an important marker for the diagnosis of injury, infection or inflammation. [55, 56] Currently, dextran-coated Fe_3O_4 FNs were used in *in vivo* applications in a pioneer magnetocardiography technique by means of Superconducting Quantum Interference Device (SQUID) gradiometry for the investigation of electromagnetic changes observed in the heart function due to hypercholesterolemia. [57]

In the present book we analyze in detail the concept of MAHD [34–37] which is based on the utilization of FNs in the conventional HD therapy in which End Stage Renal Disease (ESRD) patients have to be subjected to. The core of the idea is the production of Ferromagnetic Nanoparticles-Targeted Binding Substance Conjugates (FN-TBS Cs) constructed by FNs and a specific TBS. The TBS must have high affinity for the specific Target Toxic Substance (TTS) that should be removed from the patient during the HD session. Thus, after the FN-TBS Cs have been timely administered to the patient prior to the HD session, owing to their free circulation in the vascular network the Cs will be able to bind with the TTS through the TBS part. Consequently, the complex FN-TBS-TTS can be selectively removed during dialysis by means of a "magnetic dialyser" that is externally installed at a specific point along the extracorporeal blood circulation line of the dialysis machine. The proposed MAHD strategy offers many advantages for the patients when compared to conventional HD. These advantages are discussed among relevant technical issues in great detail. Also, while the MAHD therapy requires small investments for the modification of existing dialysis machines, it will surely offer enormous financial benefits.

For the evaluation of the MAHD concept in this book we have used Bovine Serum Albumin (BSA) as the TBS part of the Cs since it is highly biocompatible and surely improves the biocompatibility of the complete FN-BSA Cs, making them appropriate for *in vivo* applications that we believe will follow soon. However, we have also examined the possible affinity that BSA might have for specific TTSs so that the binding affinity and capacity of the complex FN-BSA Cs is improved when compared to bare FNs. Ideally, many substances such as antibodies or Human Serum Albumin (HSA) could also serve as the TBS part of the Cs. As FNs host carriers we have used Fe_2O_3/Fe_3O_4 particles owing to their relatively high biocompatibility when compared to other ferromagnetic materials. For a thorough discussion on the biocompatibility of relevant iron agents that are administered in cases of iron deficiency based anemia see Ref. [58]. As the TBS part, BSA was chosen since, except for its biocompatibility this protein has been well-studied in terms of size, shape and charge and also is commercially available in high-purity form. Thus, the Cs studied here have the specific form Fe_3O_4-BSA. Both bare Fe_3O_4 FNs and FN-BSA Cs have been studied regarding their toxin binding affinity and capacity on homocysteine, p-Cresol and β2-microglobulin. Except for the results that were obtained in the laboratory we have also performed mock-dialysis experiments on both MAHD and conventional HD where dialysers and dialysis machines that are routinely used in HD practice were employed. In these experiments homocysteine have been evaluated as a model TTS. In the

MAHD mock-dialysis experiments we used a simple "magnetic dialyser" consisting of an array of permanent magnets placed along the extracorporeal blood circulation line. All the performed experiments clearly show the *in vitro* applicability of MAHD. However, future work surely requires evaluation by means of mock-dialysis experiments on donated blood and ultimately *in vivo* applications.

The present book is structured as follows: Chapter (2) briefly reviews the most important topics related to the function of the kidney, kidney diseases and HD. Owing to the interdisciplinary character of this work such a discussion is needed in order to assist the general reader who is not familiar with these issues toward understanding their specific details. Also, this discussion will make easier understanding the advantages of MAHD over conventional HD. More specifically, Chapter (2) provides a brief discussion on the important role of the kidney in the human body, defines Chronic Kidney Disease (CKD) and addresses the most common causes that initially motivate its appearance and ultimately accelerate its evolution to ESRD. The present status of HD therapy is also reviewed. Chapter (3) introduces the proposed MAHD concept. Therein, practical issues related to MAHD are discussed and its advantages over conventional HD are presented in detail. Briefly, (i) since MAHD assists toward the selective targeting of specific toxins, prevention by disorders (for instance, renal osteodystrophy, dialysis-related amyloidosis etc) could be achieved during their early stage of evolution, (ii) decrease of HD session duration, (iii) preservation of residual renal function (RRF) etc. Chapter (4) reports on the preparation method of the specific FN-TBS Cs studied in this book, i.e. Fe_3O_4-BSA Cs and on the experimental techniques. Chapter (5) presents results on the structural/morphological and magnetic characterization of the Fe_3O_4-BSA Cs that were investigated by means of X-ray diffraction, Atomic Force Microscopy, Circular Dichroism spectropolarimetry, UV-VIS spectrophotometry, and SQUID magnetometry. Since for the realization of the MAHD concept three prerequisites are needed, namely high solubility/biocompatibility, high magnetic retraction efficiency, and high toxin binding affinity and capacity of the FN-TBS Cs, we have investigated these topics in detail. First, by means of SQUID magnetometry the magnetic retraction efficiency of the produced Cs was investigated as a function of their BSA content. Second and most important by employing Circular Dichroism spectropolarimetry, UV-VIS spectrophotometry, Nuclear Magnetic Resonance, and standard clinical methods, namely Fluorescence Polarization Immunoassay and Turbidimetry Immunoassay we have evaluated the toxin binding affinity and capacity of both bare Fe_3O_4 FNs and Fe_3O_4-BSA Cs by performing *in vitro* experiments on specific TTSs. Homocysteine, p-Cresol and β2-microglobulin were investigated in detail. Chapter (6) presents results obtained by means of both MAHD and conventional HD mock-dialysis experiments in dialysers and dialysis machines that are routinely used in HD practice. The obtained results prove the successful *in vitro* applicability of the proposed MAHD method. Finally, Chapter (7) summarizes our findings and addresses important perspectives.

Chapter 2

Hemodialysis

1. Function of Kidney

The Kidney has many basic activities in the human body. These activities could be classified in two main categories: (i) production of hormones, and (ii) filtering of unwanted blood-solute substances and their excretion into the urine. Depending on the kind of blood-solute substances that are filtered by the kidneys two subclasses should be farther distinguished in category (ii): subclasses (ii.a) and (ii.b) when the filtered substances refer to molecular and atomic ones, respectively.

(i) Briefly, the basic hormones produced by the kidney are erythropoietin, renin and an active form of vitamin D. First, erythropoietin after being produced by the kidney, is delivered to the bone marrow where it signals the production of red blood cells that, since they are necessary for the delivery of oxygen to the tissues, are probably the most basic constituent of blood. Second, renin is a hormone that actually balances blood pressure since it regulates body fluid content. Third, vitamin D regulates the balance of calcium that is the most important element for maintenance of healthy bones. Since in this book we do not deal with this first category of renal activities we will not farther discuss this subject here. We will utilize the rest of our book to the second category of kidney's activities.

(ii.a) Kidney also serves as an excellent natural filter that is able to distinguish different molecular substances among numerous ones of different molecular weight (MW), structure and atomic constituents. This natural filter should act selectively in the sense that while it should completely remove all kinds of non-biocompatible toxins from the blood, it should retain, also completely, all other elemental constituents (red blood cells, white blood cells, proteins, platelets, carbohydrates etc) since these are of primal importance for the maintenance of a perfectly functional human body. Depending on differences related to the way of their occurrence these toxins can be classified in two basic categories: (a) toxins that have been introduced in the human body *externally*, either accidentally (overdose of medical substances, under terroristic attacks etc) or on purpose (usage of drugs, suicide commitment etc), and (b) toxins that are produced by the human body *internally*. In category (a) belong all chemical substances of very common (non-steroidal anti-inflammatory substances, antibiotics, etc) or of less common (radiocontrast agents, chemical substances used in chemotherapy, etc) medical use, since such substances are mainly non-biocompatible and can affect the filtration ability of kidneys either temporarily, so that kidney function returns to baseline when these medications are discontinued, or permanently when long-term usage has already motivated partial but non-reversible vascular, tubular, interstitial or even glomerular damage. [59–61] In category (b) the related substances are those that are produced by the human body either under normal conditions, as for instance happens when ingested proteins are processed through the metabolic activities occurring mainly in the liver and muscle tissues (urea, creatinine, etc), or under abnormal processes as happens when specific proteins, that fortunately in some cases can serve as informative markers, are secreted during damage of muscle/human-organ tissues, or under inflammation conditions (C-reactive protein, serum glutamic oxaloacetic transaminase, serum glutamic pyruvic transaminase, creatine kinase, creatine phosphokinase, homocysteine, p-Cresol, etc). In this book we will deal with category (b) and specifically with the toxins that are produced during normal metabolic processes in the human body. However, the proposed MAHD strategy can be readily expanded so that substances produced during abnormal processes or even substances belonging to category (a) discussed above could also be handled.

(ii.b) Finally, kidney is responsible for the selective excretion and reabsorption of atomic substances such as minerals (potassium, sodium, calcium, phosphorous, iron, magnesium etc.) when these are in excess or in lack in the human body, respectively. Since minerals are important electrolytes in many biological processes, including both extracellular and intracellular ones, they actually modulate the functionality of all other basic organs of the human body. Thus kidney, through controlling electrolytes, practically controls the whole human body. Briefly, both potassium and calcium are of great importance for the heart functionality, so that they should be balanced at a very specific range in the blood. Also, sodium plays a very basic role in the maintenance of normal blood pressure. Finally, calcium/phosphorous balance is very important for the maintenance of a healthy skeletal system, and iron is basic for the production of healthy red blood cells.

2. Chronic Kidney Disease

Unfortunately, many parameters can influence kidney by starting at microscopic and evolving at macroscopic structural level so that its filtering ability can be gradually reduced. This situation is called Chronic Kidney Disease (CKD). Depending on the remaining filtering ability of kidney, CKD is classified in five stages. Three of the most common causes that promote CKD at a microscopic level are: (a) Hypertension, (b) Diabetes Mellitus, and (c) Hypercholesterolemia. Although Hypercholesterolemia cannot be considered as a direct cause of CKD it should not be disregarded since when it is combined with Hypertension and Diabetes Mellitus an extended disorder occurs that is related to the inadequate metabolism of proteins, carbohydrates and lipids. This disorder is known as Metabolic Syndrome.

2.1. Hypertension

Hypertension (HT) refers to the condition where high blood pressure is monitored in the vascular network of the human body. HT is commonly motivated by extended atherosclerosis of the vascular network, a condition that makes vessels to lose their elasticity. As a result, vessels cannot be dilated effectively so that high blood pressure cannot be reduced efficiently. It can easily be understood that this process will proliferate a cumulative effect; since HT cannot be counterbalanced by a damaged vascular network, in the case where anti-hypertensive medication is not timely administered the damage of the vascular network will progressively become more extended under the subjection to existing HT. Thus, although initially the local vascular network of kidney could even be normal, owing to its subjection to HT it will progressively get seriously damaged, eventually leading to CKD.

2.2. Diabetes Mellitus

Diabetes Mellitus (DM) is a second cause of equal importance to HT that can result in CKD and is related to unbalanced blood glucose levels. The cause of high blood glucose levels can be either a lack in insulin production by the pancreas, known as type-I DM, or increased resistance in muscle tissues to insulin administration, known as type-II DM. Whether it is related to type-I or type-II DM the high levels of blood glucose, when existing for prolonged times, promote atherosclerosis of the global vascular network and eventually can lead to damage of the kidney local vascular network, that is to CKD. In recent years much attention has been paid on specific substances that are so-called Advanced Glycation End Products (AGEPs). These substances result from the irreversible modification of amino acids, proteins or peptides by carbohydrates and other metabolites. In DM AGEPs predominantly result from high glucose in the blood and are associated to inflammation that could gradually result in extended atherosclerosis of the vascular network.

2.3. Hypercholesterolemia and the Metabolic Syndrome

The simultaneous occurrence of HT and DM with Hypercholesterolemia (HC) is known as the Metabolic Syndrome (MS), a term that is used to compactly describe an extended disorder of how the human-body metabolism administers proteins, carbohydrates and lipids. Owing to the improper dietary habits that our society has adopted, it is clear that today the MS is met in a wide percentage of both young and most commonly elder individuals. Fortunately, early detection and successful control of each disease that contributes to the MS will enable patients to avoid serious disorders such as CKD, coronary disease, etc. However, it should be noted that, unfortunately, CKD currently concerns an important percentage of patients having the MS. The initialization of kidney disease will farther inflict cumulative complications since kidneys are responsible for controlling blood pressure by producing hormones and regulating the body fluid content. Thus, once CKD has been initiated a progressive stage-to-stage evolution will finally lead to ESRD.

3. Hemodialysis

Depending on the remaining filtering ability of kidneys, CKD is classified in five stages, as summarized in Table 2.1. [62, 63] This quantitative classification is based on the determination of Glomerular Filtration Rate (GFR) which indicates the blood volume which is completely filtered by the glomerular capillaries per unit time. At the final stage where

Table 2.1. Classification of CKD

Stage	GFR (mL/min/1.73 m^2)
1	> 90
2	$60 - 89$
3	$30 - 59$
4	$15 - 29$
5	< 15

GFR$<$ 15 mL/min/1.73 m^2, the remaining filtering ability of kidneys is negligible. As a consequence, toxins accumulate in the patient at a rate higher than they are excreted in the urine by the kidneys. Thus, these patients, called ESRD patients, have to participate in specific renal replacement therapy which can be either HD or Peritoneal Dialysis. Although our concept could also be applicable to Peritoneal Dialysis, in this book we will exclusively refer to HD.

As shown in Figs.2.1(a)-2.1(c), during HD, the patient's blood following an extracorporeal circulation line is forced to pass through an artificial kidney, known as dialysis machine, wherein it is filtered. Generally, access to patient's blood is achieved in three different ways: (i) by an intravenous catheter that is usually placed at the internal jugular vein or at the femoral vein, (ii) by an arteriovenous fistula, and (iii) by an arteriovenous synthetic graft. In cases (ii) and (iii) an artery is joined with a vein through anastomosis at the forearm of the patient. Most commonly, access to patient's blood is achieved by using two needles that are inserted into the arteriovenous fistula at the forearm of the patient (Fig.2.1(b)). The two needles act as outlet and inlet where the blood is drawn and returned after having been filtered by the dialysis machine. Basically, the cornerstone of the dialysis machine is the dialyser wherein the blood and a balanced dialysis solution, known as the dialysate, circulate continuously in a counter-current flow that takes place into two different compartments separated by a semipermeable membrane (Fig.2.1(c)). Consequently, the semipermeable membrane allows the removal of toxins from the blood to the dialysate owing to both diffusion and convection processes. Except for the dialyser, a blood pump is mainly needed for maintaining blood circulation from the patient to the dialysis machine and back to the patient. Fortunately, owing to vast technological evolution, extra components are incorporated in every dialysis machine so that numerous parameters related to the safety of the patient are monitored automatically during the HD session. For instance, currently every state-of-the-art dialysis machine includes sensors that monitor the blood pressure and the heart rate of the patient, the blood and dialysate flow rates in the dialyser, possible air leak in the blood circulation line etc.

Nowadays, the two most important issues that concern the community of nephrologists are: (i) the initiation time, and (ii) the dose and adequacy of HD therapy. Lately, an international practice has been established for early initiation of HD therapy, especially for patients having DM, which is scheduled at three 4-hour sessions per week. It is generally believed that such a schedule delivers an adequate dose of HD to all patients. However, it is quite obvious that these issues (initiation time, dose, and adequacy of HD) cannot have a unique answer that can be applicable to every patient. Consequently, a debate currently

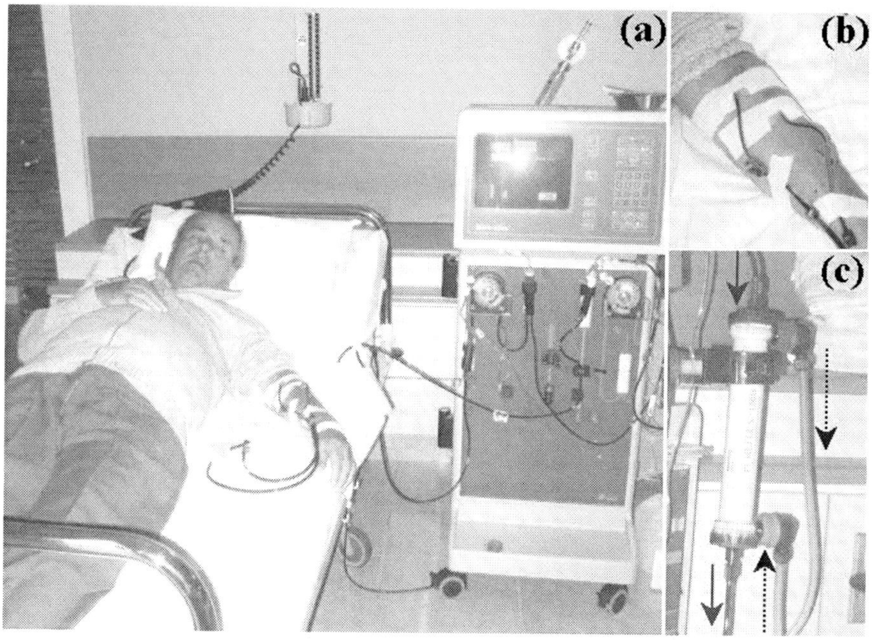

Figure 2.1. (a) During HD, blood is filtered by the dialysis machine. (b) Most commonly, access to the patient's vascular network is achieved by using two needles placed at his/her forearm. (c) Blood passes through a dialyser following an extracorporeal circulation line. In the dialyser, the blood and the dialysate circulate continuously in a counter-current flow (solid arrows: blood flow, dotted arrows: dialysate flow) that takes place into two different compartments separated by a semipermeable membrane. Toxins are removed from blood to the dialysate according to diffusion/convection physical processes. Courtesy of N. Stamopoulos.

exists on these topics.

3.1. Initiation of HD Therapy

According to recent Dialysis Outcomes Quality Initiative (DOQI) guidelines [64] it is considered that HD therapy should be started when GFR drops below approximately $10-15$ mL/min. GFR can be easily estimated by a Creatinine Clearance test, although this method results in an overestimation of $10-20\%$. More accurately, GFR can be easily estimated by using the empirical Modification-of-Diet-in-Renal-Disease (MDRD) formula GFR$=$ 186.3x(serum creatinine in mg/dL)$-$1.154x(age in years)$-$0.203x(0.742 if female)x(1.212 if patient is African American) given in Refs. [65–67] (see also Refs. [62,63]).

In the mid $80's$ Bonomini and colleagues [68] proposed that the relatively early initiation of HD therapy could prolong patient survival. Currently, an international tendency that adopts this early-initiation proposition has been established. [69–72] However, the validity of this strategy has been recently questioned [73–76] and sometimes even accused as being commercialized. Traynor and colleagues have shown that early initiation of HD fails to extend the survival of long-term-HD patients. [73] Also, Korevaar and colleagues [74] provided an alternative interpretation for the results that were originally associated with the validation of survival prolongation in the case where relatively early initiation of HD was employed. In Ref. [74] the authors demonstrated that any apparent survival benefit from relatively early initiation of HD therapy could by accounted for by the concept of the so-called lead-time bias. The lead-time bias error refers to the case where the apparent prolonged survival benefit could be due to the earlier registration of patients in the study. [73–76]

3.2. Dose and Adequacy of HD Therapy

Most commonly, nephrologists evaluate the adequacy of HD dose by estimating the Urea Reduction Ratio (URR) given by the simple expression URR=$[(U_{in}-U_{fin})/U_{in}]$x100%, where U_{in} and U_{fin} are the predialysis and postdialysis urea levels. A value of 65% per session is the recommended target. However, due to strong criticism, in recent years the URR parameter has been replaced by the Kt/V criterion, where K is the nominal urea clearance of the dialyser (provided by the manufacturer), t is the duration of a HD session, and V is the patient fluid volume. In this criterion the minimum target value recommended per session equals 1.2. As was indicated by HEMO study, no significant improvement in outcome was observed when the single pool Kt/V referring to urea was increased from 1 .25 to 1.65. [77–79] Recently, the so-called HD Product (HDP) defined as HDP=(hours per HD session)x(HD sessions per week) has also been introduced for evaluating the adequacy of HD therapy on a weekly basis. [80]

3.3. HD Schedule Customized to Each ESRD Patient

The discussion made here reveals that fundamental issues related to ESRD and HD therapy are still under intense clinical studies that try to remove existing controversies. In our opinion the existence of such controversies is not surprising since these subjects are quite complex owing to the many parameters that are getting involved. Owing to the complex function of kidneys, in each patient CKD gradually evolves to ESRD by following one of many different pathways. Also, specific personal health problems such as coronary heart disease that is usually met in clinical practice, or other cardiovascular problems (congestive heart failure, left ventricular dysfunction, etc) should be considered and carefully evaluated. Thus, although currently there is a clear tendency for an all-cases-applicable HD schedule, a customized therapy that could be tailored to the exact needs of each patient should ideally be the desired aim.

In order to stress the need for a more customized HD therapy and to make easier the connection to the MAHD strategy, some of the specific discrete cases that are met in clinical practice are briefly discussed here. As a first general example we mention that in some cases the kidneys do not lose their filtering ability for all substances at the same time. Most commonly, as CKD evolves to ESRD the kidneys can retain their ability to efficiently filter some toxic substances, while they are completely unable to handle others. Thus, at least generally speaking, a patient could be bound to participate HD therapy owing to impaired renal function for only a few toxic substances. Second, even when CKD is associated with improper control of many toxic substances, in some cases the kidneys exhibit pronounced unbalance of some specific substances, a condition that could inflict serious implications. These implications could be intense, eventually leading to high morbidity and mortality, in cases when these strongly unbalanced substances are of high toxicity. For instance, today there is no reliable evidence that urea, a molecular substance that traditionally serves as a basic marker for evaluating the adequacy of HD dose, is actually related to toxicity. [18–22, 81] Thus, in recent years it has been recognized that although urea, which has low MW of 60 D, can serve as a representative marker for other substances of comparable MW (MW$<$ 500 D), it cannot be reliably used for estimating the filtering of other toxic substances that either have significantly higher MW (for instance, β2-microglobulin having MW= 11.818 D, leptin having MW= 16.000 D, and other AEGPs), or of substances that although they can have MW comparable to urea, they have an affinity to bound with proteins (for instance, homocysteine having MW= 135 D, and p-Cresol having MW= 108 D). [18–22] The transport dynamics of these substances are diffusion limited in semipermeable membranes having pores of small size as the ones that are currently used in dialysers. [78, 82] Thus, the accumulation of middle-MW substances such as β2-microglobulin can result in serious disorders. HEMO study [79] revealed that the increased removal of relatively larger molecules -as represented by β2-microglobulin- is associated with less cardiovascular mortality, the leading cause of death for patients on HD. [83] Contrasting to the unsubstantiated toxicity of urea, it is well known that potassium, an atomic toxic substance, inflicts a pronounced toxicity owing to the direct impact that it has on heart function. Thus, although potassium should be carefully balanced in all patients on HD therapy, special care should be taken in individuals who have extra heart problems. Also, one of the protein-bound substances, that as has been shown exerts a substantial impact on biological systems, is p-Cresol. [84, 85] Thus, this specific substance should be carefully balanced. Finally, as a more specific case we report the way of action of β2-microglobulins. It is well known that in patients participating in chronic HD therapy a special disorder called dialysis-related amyloidosis is almost unavoidable. [28, 29] This disorder refers to the case when molecules of β2-microglobulin join together forming large complexes that have the form of chains, the so-called amyloids. [28–30, 86–90] These large complexes cannot be removed by using conventional dialysers, so they ultimately deposit in organs, joints, and tendons, interfering with their normal function. [28–30, 86–90]

From the discussion made above it is clear that, ideally, each ESRD patient should follow a customized HD schedule adjacent to his/her specific needs. This will provide maximum comfort with minimum morbidity, eventually offering a better quality-of-life to the patient. The flexible MAHD strategy that we propose in this book could assist to this end, since it can be adjusted to the exact requirements of each patient.

Chapter 3

Magnetically Assisted Hemodialysis

The method that we propose as an evolution of conventional HD is termed as MAHD [see Refs. [34–37] and http://nanotechweb.org/cws/article/lab/32024] and is based on the following concept: Under the application of an external magnetic field, at a collection point that could be placed either at the dialyser or at another point of the blood circulation line, the efficient removal of toxic substances can be easily achieved once these are bound to FN-TBS Cs that are timely administered to the patient prior to the HD session. A complex FN-TBS-TTS is schematically shown in Fig.3.1.

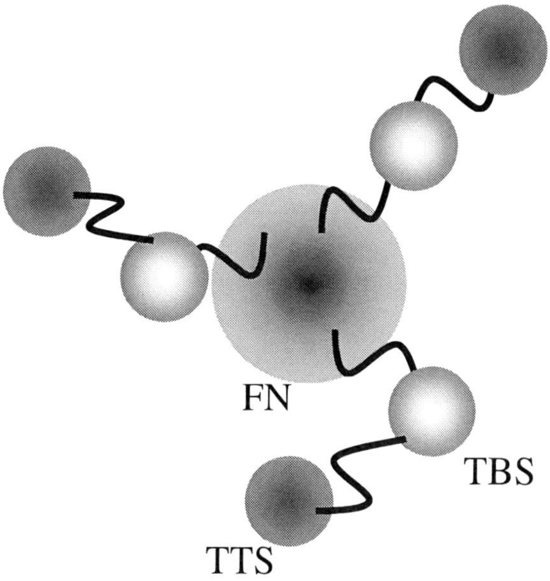

Figure 3.1. The concept of Magnetically Assisted Hemodialysis is based on the production of FN-TBS Cs that have high affinity for a specific TTS. Specific proteins and antibodies could serve as TBSs. After these FN-TBS Cs are administered to the patient, they will bind with the TTS owing to their free circulation in the vascular network. Consequently, the TTS that are bound to the FN-TBS Cs can be easily retracted during dialysis by means of a "magnetic dialyser" (see Fig.3.2).

A detailed discussion that illuminates this concept is made here. The core of the idea is the production of Cs constructed by FNs and a specifically designed TBS. The TBS must have high affinity for a specific TTS. In many cases antibodies could serve as the TBS part of the FN-TBS Cs. Also, simple proteins could serve as TBSs since many middle-MW toxins have high affinity for specific proteins. We note that antibodies for some of the TTSs (for instance, creatinine antibodies) have been developed not only for research purposes [91] but, hopefully are already commercially available. [92] The FN-TBS Cs should be dissolved in a host solution that should be both stable and biocompatible. Thus, once the FN-TBS Cs have been administered to the patient they will be able to bind with the desired TTS owing to their free circulation in the bloodstream. The administration of the FN-TBS Cs should be done timely prior to the MAHD session so that enough time will be provided for the efficient binding with the TTS. Consequently, the complex FN-TBS-TTS can be selectively removed by a "magnetic dialyser" that is a magnetic-field device applied either directly at the conventional dialyser or at a different point along the extracorporeal blood circulation line. The "magnetic dialyser" should be designed so as to provide intense magnetic-field gradients that are necessary to immobilize the FNs and eventually the TTS that is bound onto them. The proposed strategy is schematically presented in Fig.3.2.

1. Practical Issues Related to MAHD

A number of practical issues related to the MAHD strategy are discussed here: [34,35]

1.1. Biocompatibility/Solubility

The FN-TBS Cs should be absolutely biocompatible in order to avoid serious conflicts with the immune system. Also, the Cs must be perfectly saline soluble so that possible precipitation and subsequent thrombotic complications are avoided. To this end, for successful *in vivo* applications the coating of the FNs surface with a completely biocompatible/soluble substance (proteins, carbohydrates or lipids) is a necessity. In a late stage, biocompatible, however indigestible substances should be considered as coating so that the duration of their circulation in the vascular network will be maximized.

1.2. Way of Administration

The administration of the FN-TBS Cs can be done easily by an intravenous injection. This is the routine practice in all *in vivo* applications. However, for ESRD patients on HD the preservation of a healthy vascular network in the regime were needle access is routinely performed is a very important issue. Most importantly for this reason, but also for reasons of patient's comfort, the preferable way of administration would ultimately be the ingestion of the FN-TBS Cs via the gastrointestinal tract. For this reason increased attention on the biocompatibility of the FN-TBS Cs should be paid since absorption through the gastrointestinal tract inevitably follows the liver tract wherein intense phagocytic action could lead not only to the temporal miss of the goal but also to permanent liver disorders. As mentioned above, biocompatibility is the most crucial issues in this case: appropriately

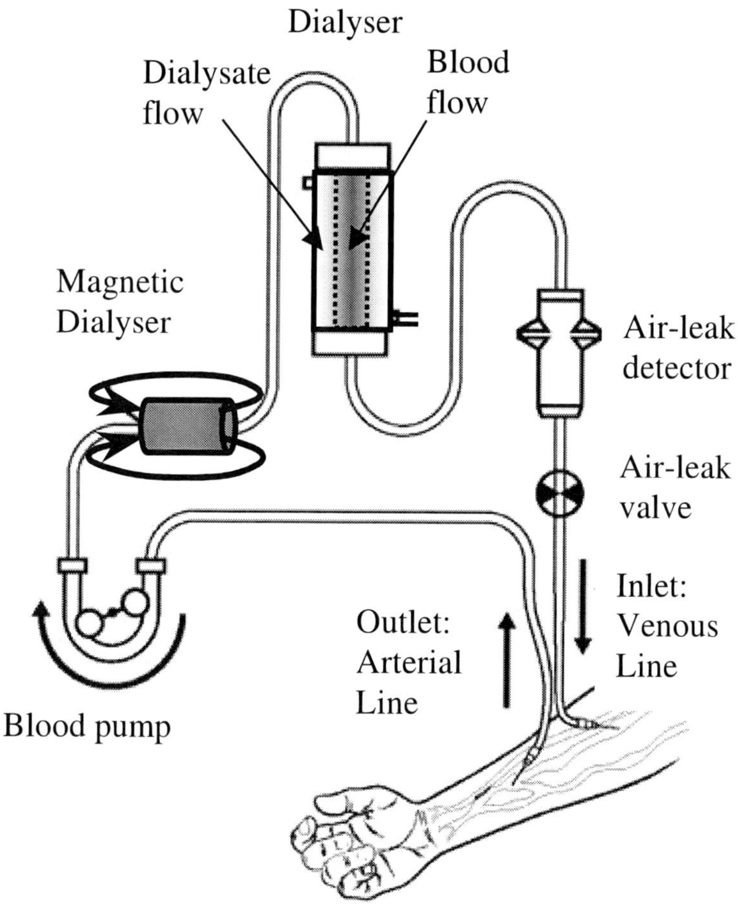

Figure 3.2. The concept of Magnetically Assisted Hemodialysis is schematically presented. Apart from the standard automatically controlled components that are used for maintaining the blood and dialysate counter-current flows and additional detectors that are used for monitoring numerous parameters related to the safety of the patient, a "magnetic dialyser" that provides intense magnetic-field gradients is applied directly at the conventional dialyser or at another point of the extracorporeal blood circulation line. The "magnetic dialyser" retracts the FN-TBS-TTS Cs so that after only a few blood iterations the TTS is removed from the patient.

biocompatible, however indigestible substances should be mostly considered for coating the FNs surface so that the duration of their circulation in the vascular network is maximized.

1.3. Patient Friendly Method

It should be stressed that the proposed MAHD method is non-invasive. We recall that the presence of FN-TBS Cs in the patient body is only transient since they will be removed entirely at the end of each MAHD session. This should be a prerequisite, since even in the case where the employed FNs are completely biocompatible even extremely small quantities that could remain after sequential MAHD sessions would progressively lead to serious liver disorders. Finally, in the case where, hopefully, FN-TBS Cs appropriate for administration through the gastrointestinal tract are designed, the patient would experience great comfort.

1.4. Synergetic Applicability of MAHD with Conventional HD

The proposed MAHD strategy that relies on the magnetically assisted indirect retraction of toxin substances does not oppose to conventional HD therapy that relies on exchange of toxins through diffusion/convection physical processes. At both an early experimental stage and at a following stage of clinical trials both techniques could be employed in parallel.

1.5. Magnetic Retraction Efficiency and Toxin Binding Affinity and Capacity

In order to have adequate magnetic retraction efficiency of the Cs at the "magnetic dialyser" two main prerequisites should be fulfilled: First, the FN-TBS Cs should be highly magnetic. Second, the "magnetic dialyser" should produce intense magnetic-field gradients. Furthermore, the successful applicability of MAHD is ultimately based on a third prerequisite: the Cs should have high binding affinity and capacity for the respective TTS. Thus, the host carriers FNs should be fully covered with the respective TBS. These very important issues and some underlying conflicts are discussed in detail in Chapter (5).

2. Advantages of MAHD over Conventional HD

The advantages of MAHD in comparison to conventional HD should be clarified here: [34–37]

2.1. Selective Targeting and Prevention by Disorders during Early Stages

As was discussed above, not all, but specific toxic substances play a crucial role for the health status of long-term-HD patients. In contrast to the solute toxins of small MW (such as urea which has MW=60 D), the removal of specific middle-MW substances such as β2-microglobulin or other protein-bound molecules such as homocycteine is very important for the overall health status of the patient. *Thus, at least at a very early stage, our method could be employed for the selective removal of such TTS of high biological importance.*

As a first example we mention the disorder of dialysis-related amyloidosis that is related to the existence of increased blood-serum levels of β2-microglobulin. [28, 29] These β2-microglobulin molecules have the tendency to bind together forming extended structures, called fibrils, that cannot be removed by using conventional dialysers. These fibrils ultimately deposit in organs, joints, and tendons interfering with their normal function. [28–30, 86–90] The design of FN-TBS Cs that will exclusively bind to β2-microglobulin molecules would enable the maintenance of normal blood-serum levels and prevention from dialysis-related amyloidosis. Also, TBSs that bind directly to fibrils could be employed for the removal of already formed ones.

As a second example, our method could be a possible candidate for the rapid removal of target atomic substances such as electrolytes. It is well known that in severe episodes, extremely elevated potassium levels can even become the first cause of death mainly by motivating inherent cardiovascular abnormalities. In such cases the typical clinical approach relies on simultaneous intravenous injection of a diuretic substance and a counterbalanced solution which is compatible to blood serum. However, in severe episodes this conventional approach could be time-consuming and eventually inefficient, leading to high mortality. The use of specific FN-TBS Cs could significantly reduce the time needed for the removal of extra amounts of the specific electrolyte during a single MAHD session.

Our work eventually aims to the construction of a Multi Targeted Binding Substance (MTBS) which will be able to bind with many TTSs (creatinine, urea, homocysteine, β2-microglobulin etc). Thus, ultimately a small amount of FN-MTBS Cs will be required in order to remove as many toxic substances as possible during a single MAHD session. Fig.3.3 schematically presents the ideal MTBS.

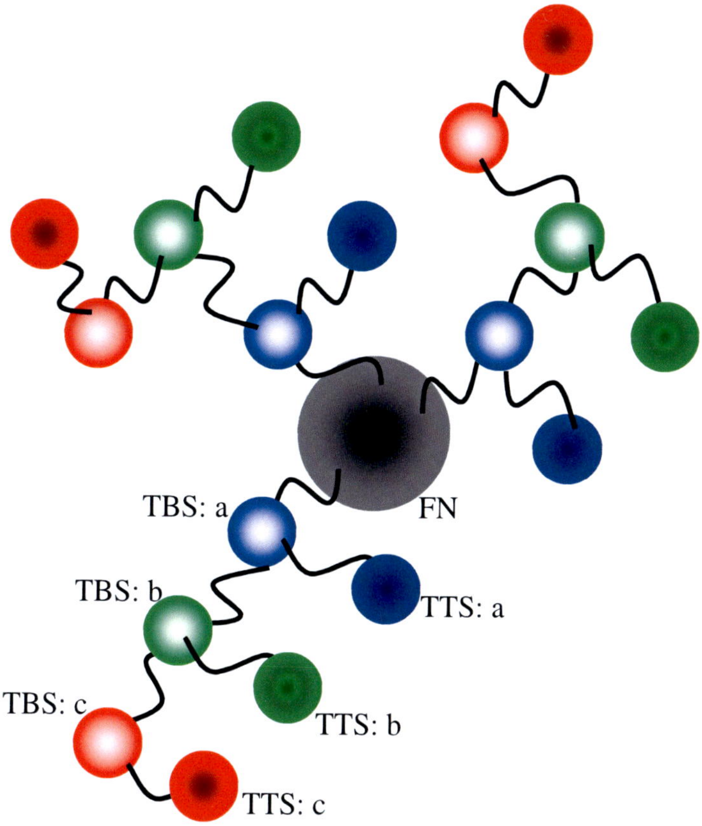

Figure 3.3. Magnetically Assisted Hemodialysis that is based on FN-MTBS Cs is the ultimate goal of the proposed concept. Various proteins and antibodies should be attached to the surface of a FN. Thus, such Cs could effectively remove almost all toxins from the patient [Reproduced from Ref. [34]].

2.2. Decrease of HD Session Duration

Since the FN-TBS Cs will be administered timely prior to the MAHD session, their efficient binding with the respective TTS and the subsequent retraction of the complex FN-TBS-TTS by the "magnetic dialyser" will allow the complete removal of the TTS in only a few iterations of blood circulation. This should be contrasted to conventional HD where the exchange of toxins between the blood and dialysate takes place *during* the session and is determined by the dynamics of the diffusion/convection physical processes. This makes conventional HD a rather insufficient, time-consuming technique wherein the whole blood of the patient must accomplish many complete iterations in order for adequate HD dose to be succeeded. For instance, by assuming a blood flow rate in the dialyser of 250 mL/min and that the body blood content is approximately 8% of the total body weight, we conclude that in a 4-hour HD session approximately 10 complete iterations of blood circulation are accomplished for an 80 Kg patient. In contrast, in the proposed strategy the binding of the FN-TBS Cs to the TTS has already been achieved *prior* to the actual MAHD session. Thus, during MAHD the TTS are ready to get retracted by the "magnetic dialyser" owing to their binding with the FNs through the TBS constituent. *We believe that this would lead to a pronounced decrease of each MAHD session duration.* Obviously, this would be a great advantage for the patient.

2.3. Adjustment of the Blood Flow Rate

As discussed above, MAHD enables the more efficient removal of toxins so that the duration of each dialysis session could be strikingly reduced. However, MAHD offers an additional opportunity especially for the cases where the standard 4-hour duration session is still preferable. Owing to the significantly higher rate of toxin removal per blood circulation, the necessary iterations for a 4-hour MAHD session should be significantly lower than the ones needed for a 4-hour conventional HD session for the same target dialysis dose to be delivered to the patient. Thus, since in a 4-hour MAHD session we are able to achieve the target dialysis dose with lower blood-circulation iterations, we have the opportunity to *selectively employ a lower blood flow rate.* Depending on the hemodynamic status of the patient the blood flow rate usually employed during HD ranges in 200 – 300 mL/min. Using even lower blood flow rates could be of great importance for patients who have intense cardiovascular problems.

Ultimately, the MAHD strategy offers the opportunity to choose the most appropriate values for the two basic parameters that determine the dose and adequacy of the delivered dialysis, that is the session duration and the blood flow rate. This will allow the construction of a flexible MAHD schedule that will offer to the patient maximum comfort without being burdensome to his/her specific health problems.

2.4. Preservation of Residual Renal Function

As discussed until now the introduction of MAHD could enable the substantiation of customized HD schedules tailored to the exact needs of each individual. For instance, as it was discussed above, as ESRD is progressively established only a couple of toxic substances could be seriously unbalanced. Thus, instead of the patient being subjected to typical HD, the administration of the FN-TBS Cs that are relative to the few unbalanced TTSs could allow their selective removal. More importantly, as already discussed above, MAHD would enable minimization of each HD session duration. This in turn would surely assist the preservation of (residual renal function) RRF for longer times after initiation of HD. [93–95] Since kidneys efficiently filter toxic substances of middle MW and also protein-bound substances that cannot be removed during conventional HD, the preservation of RRF is an important issue for the overall health status of the patient. It is known that the decline of RRF aggravates during HD, [93–95] thus providing a minimum, however adequate, dialysis dose will surely assist the preservation of RRF. Consequently, owing to the preservation of RRF, initiation of the typical schedule of conventional HD (three 4-hour sessions per week) could be shifted to *much later times* when anuria is eventually established. It is obvious that this would improve both patient's comfort and overall health status.

However, we stress that when anuria (the condition in which the kidneys of a patient do not produce urine) is established, the typical HD schedule (three 4-hour sessions per week) is usually inevitable. Extra fluids that accumulate in the patient body should be removed during HD by ultrafiltration, thus targeting the so-called "dry weight" at the end of each session. [96, 97] This is accomplished by adjusting the hydrostatic pressure between the blood and the dialysate compartments of the dialyser so that the desired amount of water progressively moves from the former to the latter. Since hypotensive events should be avoided, safety reasons demand the removal of extra fluids to be mildly accomplished at the lowest possible rate (see Ref. [98] and references therein). Patients who have significant interdialytic weight gain, thus significantly exceeding their "dry weight" have to be subjected to dialysis sessions of increased duration. In such cases the session duration of MAHD cannot be shortened. However, patients who slightly exceed their "dry weight" can be subjected to shorter dialysis sessions, thus benefiting from MAHD.

2.5. Financial Benefits and Costs for Modulating Existing Dialysis Machines

The decrease of each MAHD session duration that was discussed above would permit the more efficient management of already existing Dialysis Units. More patients would be able to participate in the case when, formerly, constraints on the resources inhibited their adequate therapy. The decrease of each MAHD session's duration would also decrease the financial costs that are spent on related personnel, maintenance of dialysis machines, etc. Finally, the costs needed for the modulation of existing dialysis machines is negligible. The only serious modification is the installation of an external "magnetic dialyser" either directly at the conventional dialyser or at another point of the extracorporeal blood circulation line. In both cases, modified blood circulation lines are only needed that have an extra small compartment which should allow the retraction of FN-TBS-TTS so that the flow of the blood is not affected.

2.6. Selective Targeting of Toxic Substances that Are Administered Externally

Finally, we briefly mention the possible applicability of MAHD for toxic substances that are not produced *internally* through the normal functions of human metabolism but are introduced *externally* either by accident or on purpose (overdose of medicines, under terrorist attacks, usage of drugs, suicide attempts etc). Given that FN-TBS Cs that are relative to the externally administered specific TTS is commercially available, MAHD could be employed. In such cases, MAHD could significantly reduce the time needed for the complete removal of the toxic substance, so that it could eventually be proven as an efficient life-saving modality.

2.7. Prospects Related to Research Issues in Nephrology

We have to stress that apart from the great benefits that the proposed MAHD strategy could offer to ESRD patients, the method could also designate a new pathway regarding basic research issues in Nephrology. For instance, despite the great technological advances in diagnostic/imaging techniques and the vast amount of knowledge related to biochemical/biomedical issues, controversies still exist regarding the toxicity of various candidate substances that are related, sometimes even undocumented, to the so-called uremic syndrome. The uremic syndrome is related to the retention of numerous solute substances in the patient blood in amounts that significantly exceed the normal concentrations that are met in healthy individuals. However, even in the case when a substance is met in significantly high levels in an uremic patient, this does not directly prove its toxicity. The toxicity of an uremic substance is fairly documented when high blood-serum levels of this substance exert a detrimental action on specific organs, i.e. regarding their function, clear symptoms are observed that should disappear when its blood-serum levels go back to normal (for further information on these topics see Refs. [18–22]).

The synergetic effect of candidate toxic substances can also be investigated by employing MAHD. In some cases, although each substance of a collection of candidate ones cannot be considered as being toxic, the synergy of these substances can result in intense uremic syndrome. For instance, a long time ago it was shown in *in vivo* applications that high blood-serum levels of either urea, creatinine, guanidinosuccinic acid or methyl-guanidine do not exert significant influence on heart function. In contrast, the coexistence of high blood-serum levels of all four substances has a relatively strong impact, since it causes depression in cardiac output and coronary flow. [99] Until now we did not have a reliable way to remove specific toxins from uremic patients. MAHD enables us to *selectively decrease* the blood-serum levels of specific toxins so that the action of each one of them is evaluated. We note that another way to evaluate the possible toxicity of a substance in ESRD patients would be to *selectively increase* the blood-serum levels of the substance by gradually adding this substance to the patient. However, this protocol is unethical and should be rejected *a priori*. For instance, let us refer to the case of a substance that both low- and high-flux dialysers cannot remove. In order to study the possible toxicity of this substance by following the *selectively increase* protocol we would have to subject ESRD patients to significant risk without being able to restore the substance's blood-serum levels back to normal. In contrast, by employing MAHD we are able to adopt the *selectively decrease* protocol that restores the otherwise increased blood-serum levels of the substance. In this way not only indications but uncontested evidence can be drawn regarding the toxicity of each candidate substance.

Chapter 4

Preparation of FN-TBS Cs and Experimental Details

1. Materials

All chemicals were reagent grade and were used as such unless otherwise noted. Iron(II)chloride tetrahydrate ($FeCl_2 \cdot 4H_2O$, ReagentPlus, 99%), iron(III)chloride ($FeCl_3$, reagent grade, 97%), Urea (ACS reagent, 99%), creatinine (anhydrous), D,L-homocysteine [> 95% (titration)], p-Cresol (99%) and iron(II,III)oxide, nanopowder (98 + %) were purchased from Aldrich. Human β2-microglobulin [> 98%] was purchased from ProSpec. Bovine serum albumin, Fraction V (minimum 96%, lyophilized powder) was purchased from SIGMA. Analytical grade NH_4OH was purchased from AnalytiCals (Carlo Erba). Water was purified by analytical-grade water purification systems (Millipore). Sodium chloride for injection (Fresenius, 0.9% w/v) was purchased from a local pharmacy.

2. Preparation of Samples

In many cases the preparation of relative Cs relies on the initial production of the FNs, their subsequent *surface modification*, and finally the attachment of the desired biological substance on the *modified* surface of the host carriers. However, in this way the produced Cs cannot be sufficiently biocompatible owing to the chemical treatment that they were subjected to.

In our work, in order to increase the biocompatibility of the produced FN-TBS Cs we preferred to keep their chemical treatment to a minimum. This will be important for our *in vivo* applications that we hope will follow in the near future. Thus, we tried to conjugate the FNs with the TBS without using extra mediators. We have chosen Fe_3O_4 as the host carrier FNs and BSA as the TBS part since these two constituents are both biocompatible and have been studied in great detail in the literature regarding their structural/morphological and physical properties. [52, 53, 100–103] The employed BSA has a twofold purpose: (a) to make the Fe_3O_4 FNs more biocompatible and (b) to possibly act as a TBS of high affinity for specific TTSs.

Referring to the preparation process of the Fe_3O_4-BSA Cs we note that in our method we have used BSA as a *host environment* where the preparation of the Fe_3O_4 FNs takes place. This means that BSA is dissolved either in ultrapure water or saline, then the constituents were added, that is anhydrous $FeCl_3$ and $FeCl_2 \cdot 4H_2O$, so that the preparation of the Fe_2O_3/Fe_3O_4 FNs is carried out by chemical co-precipitation without any additional chemical constituents. More specifically, the preparation was routinely achieved by mixing 40.5 mg (0.25 mmol) anhydrous $FeCl_3$ (MW 160.20) and 49.7 mg (0.25 mmol) $FeCl_2 \cdot 4H_2O$ (MW 198.81) in the BSA host solution of ultrapure water or saline. Subsequently, the complete precipitation of the Fe_2O_3/Fe_3O_4 FNs was achieved by the abrupt addition of NH_4OH (1.5 mL, $NH_4OH{:}H_2O$ 1 : 2) to the suspension eventually reaching pH$= 9 - 9.5$. The vials were immediately sealed, to avoid exposure to atmospheric O_2 and were either mildly stirred or were subjected to intense vortex stirring. *This procedure leads to the simultaneous adsorption of BSA onto the produced FNs carriers.* Experiments were carried out at different temperatures, ranging from 2 ^oC to 50 ^oC, and different BSA concentrations of 0.5 mg/mL - 10 mg/mL of the host solution in order to examine how the BSA content of the Cs and subsequently their properties are influenced.

3. Experimental Techniques

The detailed magnetic characterization of both bare FNs and FN-TBS Cs was performed by means of a superconducting quantum interference device (SQUID) magnetometer (Quantum Design). The X-ray diffraction (XRD) spectra were collected with a SIEMENS D500 powder diffractometer using Cu-Ka radiation. Atomic Force Microscopy (AFM) images were obtained by means of a NT-MDT Solver PRO scanning probe microscope. A Circular Dichroism (CD) spectropolarimeter [Jasco J715 ($180 - 900$ nm) with incorporated an automated Peltier temperature controller] was used for evaluating the conjugation between FNs and TBSs and estimating the thermal stability of TBS protein. A UV-VIS spectrophotometer [SHIMADZU UV2100 ($200 - 900$ nm)] was also used for evaluating the conjugation between FNs and TBSs and also for estimating the toxin binding capacity of the produced FN-TBS Cs. Two Nuclear Magnetic Resonance (NMR) spectrometers of 250 MHz and 500 MHz [Bruker AC 250 MHz and Avance DRX 500 MHz] were used for the structural characterization and also for estimating the toxin binding capacity of the produced FN-TBS Cs. Standard clinical methods have also been employed, namely Fluorescence Polarization Immunoassay (FPIA) and Turbidimetry Immunoassay (TIA) for the quantitative determination of homocysteine and β2-microglobulin, respectively. These methods are routinely used in clinical practice and were feasible by employing two Abbott platforms, namely AxSYM and AEROSET®, respectively. Finally, a conventional stereoscope [LEICA, MZ6] was employed for the visual inspection of dialysers that were used in the mock-dialysis experiments.

Chapter 5

Experimental Results Obtained in the Laboratory

As discussed above the utilization of candidate FN-BSA Cs in the MAHD [34–37] concept is based on three main prerequisites: First, high biocompatibility/solubility that will guarantee their free circulation in the vascular network. Second, strong magnetic susceptibility that will enable their easy retraction at the collection point of the extracorporeal blood circulation line where the "magnetic dialyser" is applied. Third, high binding affinity and capacity of the FN-TBS Cs with the TTSs.

Thus, in this section we discuss in detail these requirements for the specific Fe_3O_4-BSA Cs employed in this book. Firstly, we discuss the structural/morphological and magnetic characterization of these Cs. The modification of both their solubility and their magnetic character on the various parameters that interfere during their preparation process are also discussed. Subsequently, we performed *in vitro* experiments for evaluating both their magnetic retraction efficiency and most importantly their binding affinity and capacity for specific toxins.

1. Structure/Morphology and Magnetism of the FN-BSA Cs

In Figs.5.1(a)-5.1(b) we show representative XRD data for bare Fe_2O_3/Fe_3O_4 FNs (no BSA adsorbed) as prepared in this book, in comparison to commercial ones. Commercial Fe_2O_3/Fe_3O_4 FNs (Aldrich) were obtained in order to be examined as an alternative candidate for the purposes of this work. However, finally we exclusively employed the homemade FNs owing to their better magnetic properties. The diffraction peaks obtained for the homemade FNs are relatively broad (5.1(a)) when compared to the respective ones obtained for commercial FNs (5.1(b)). This is probably motivated by their comparatively smaller size.

The diffraction pattern of our homemade FNs exhibit less peaks when compared to the commercial material. The extra peaks that are observed in the commercial FNs (indicated by the vertical dotted lines) can be safely ascribed to the existence of Fe_2O_3 nanoparticles.

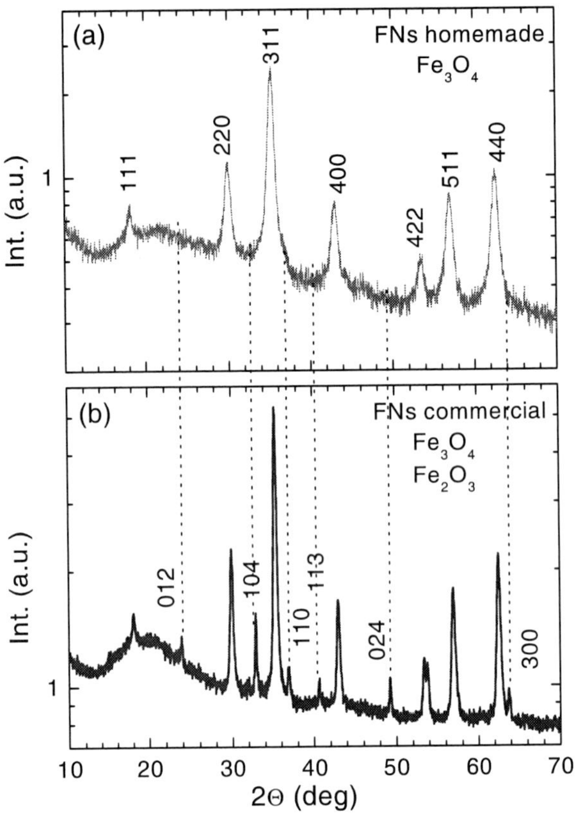

Figure 5.1. XRD data for homemade (a) and commercial (b) Fe_2O_3/Fe_3O_4 FNs. The homemade FNs mostly consist of Fe_3O_4, while the commercial ones contain significant amounts of Fe_2O_3 material. The extra peaks that are only observed in the commercial FNs, indicated by the vertical dotted lines, can be safely ascribed to Fe_2O_3 material.

After a careful analysis of the diffraction peaks observed in the homemade FNs we conclude that these peaks almost exclusively refer to the formation of Fe_3O_4 rather than Fe_2O_3. Generally, the diffraction peaks that are related to Fe_2O_3 and Fe_3O_4 materials exhibit small 2Θ displacements making the distinction between Fe_2O_3 and Fe_3O_4 quite difficult. However, in the case of the homemade FNs a close inspection and comparison with the relevant XRD database reveals that the obtained diffraction peaks can be safely ascribed to the almost exclusive formation of Fe_3O_4. In contrast, the commercial FNs constitute of both Fe_2O_3 and Fe_3O_4 in comparable amounts. Thus, owing to the higher magnetic susceptibility of Fe_3O_4 when compared to Fe_2O_3 we used the homemade FNs for our purposes. However, this detail is not crucial. Generally, any ferromagnetic material that in the form of small FNs fulfills the basic requirements of biocompatibility/solubility and relatively strong magnetic susceptibility could serve equally well for the MAHD concept discussed in this book.

Figure 5.2 shows a representative AFM image of bare Fe_3O_4 FNs (no BSA adsorbed). In order for the AFM technique to successfully reveal the Fe_3O_4 FNs, we followed a specific procedure for the preparation of the samples to be imaged: after adequate dispersion, a drop of Fe_3O_4 FNs was deposited on a silicon substrate that was formerly cleansed by means of

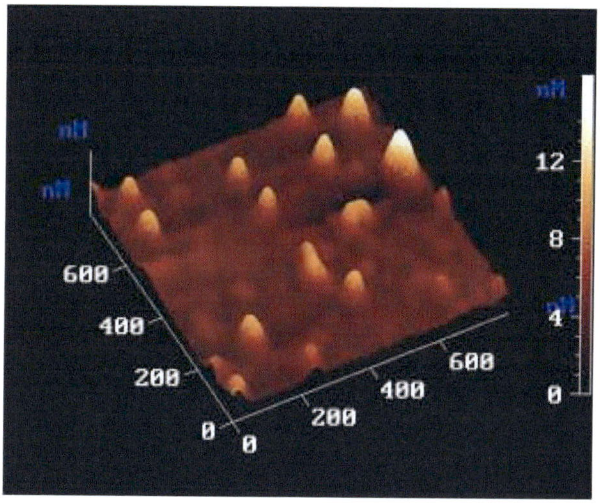

Figure 5.2. A representative AFM image of bare Fe_3O_4 FNs. The size of the specific FNs ranges between 50 – 200 nm. Statistical analysis results in a mean value of approximately 60 – 120 nm for the size of the FNs. This mean value depends on the exact preparation conditions.

sonication in an ethanol or acetone bath. We observe that the Fe_3O_4 FNs exhibit a rather big size that ranges in 50 – 200 nm. Statistical analysis of the obtained AFM images revealed that the size distribution of bare FNs has mean value that ranges in 60 – 120 nm. Both the size distribution and the mean size value depend on the specific preparation conditions.

At first sight this rather big size of FNs could be considered as a disadvantage. For instance, such a big size can inhibit their efficient intracellular delivery. However, our purposes rely on the free circulation of FNs in the vascular network and their efficient retraction by means of a "magnetic dialyser" that is installed at the dialysis machine. The homemade FNs are appropriate for these two purposes. First, their relatively big size does not inhibit their free circulation in the vascular network (typical dimensions of arteries/veins are in the range of cm to μm). Second, this rather big size guaranties their high magnetic susceptibility since the superparamagnetic limit [52] is avoided; when the size of FNs decreases below a few decades nm their saturation magnetization degrades so that extremely small FNs cannot be susceptible to easy manipulation by means of a relatively moderate magnetic field. Also, even in the case where we are well above the superparamagnetic limit the capture magnetic force experienced by a FN depends on its volume. Thus, larger FNs are captured more efficiently. Indeed, in Ref. [104] it was nicely shown that a magnetic field applied at a microvessel wherein Fe_3O_4 FNs flow, can only retract particles of size *exceeding a critical value.* Depending on the specific value of the magnetic field, the critical lower dimension of the FNs that is obtained in Ref. [104] is in the range of a few hundred nm. A couple of other reasons which advocate that FNs of rather big size as the ones studied in this book are probably imperative for the substantiation of MAHD should be noted as well. First, extremely small FNs could be subjected to increased renal clearance (see Ref. [105, 106] and references therein) before achieving the desired purpose. Second, and most important it is well known that for the case of carbohydrate-coated iron nanoparticle agents that are administered for assisting erythropoiesis, the lower the overall MW and size of the conjugate agent (ranging in 38 – 265 kD and 3 – 30 nm, respectively for the different carbohydrates that are employed as coating) the more rapid its clearance from the plasma after an intravenous dose is administered. [58] Thus, we can assume that even bigger FNs, as the ones studied in this book, could be appropriate for achieving high circulation durations that are needed for the realization of the MAHD concept.

The observation of the Fe_3O_4-BSA Cs structure with the AFM technique was not possible. This is not surprising since BSA molecules have an effective radius of approximately 3.5 nm when folded. [107] Even in the unfolded state the effective radius of BSA does not exceed 8 nm. [107, 108] The AFM technique is not so sensitive to resolve a 3.5 – 8 nm molecule that is adsorbed on a 60 – 120 nm FN.

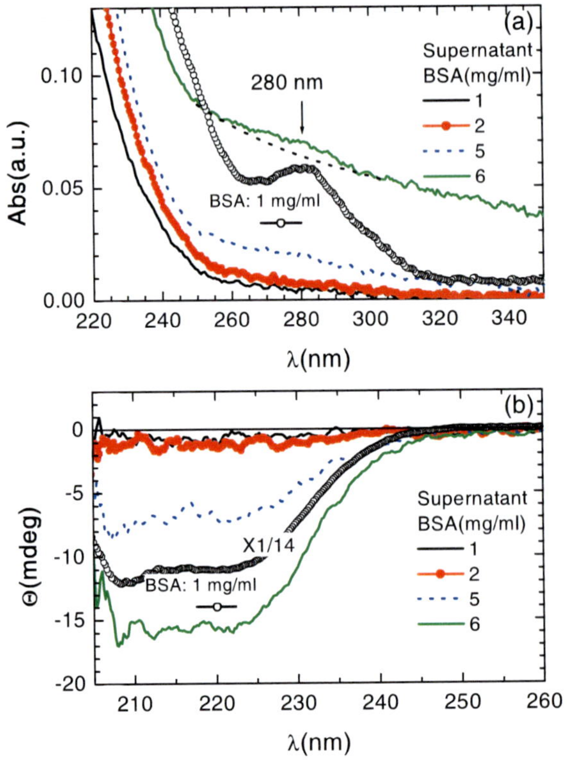

Figure 5.3. (a) UV-VIS (focused in the range of 220 – 350 nm) and (b) CD data for the supernatant of the Fe_3O_4-BSA Cs that were prepared under rigorous vortex stirring at $T_{reac} = 25\ ^oC$ for BSA concentrations of 1, 2, 5, and 6 mg/mL of the host solution. The supernatant samples were collected while the formed Cs were trapped by means of an external magnetic field. In both sets of data the respective curves of a reference BSA solution of concentration 1 mg/mL are also shown.

However, the conjugation between the Fe_3O_4 FNs and BSA molecules can be reliably proven by means of both CD spectropolarimetry and UV-VIS spectrophotometry. In Figs.5.3(a)-5.3(b) we present comparative UV-VIS and CD data respectively, that were obtained for FN-BSA Cs prepared under rigorous vortex stirring at $T_{reac} = 25\ ^oC$ for various

BSA concentrations of the host solution. These data refer to the supernatant samples that were collected when the formed Cs were trapped by means of an external magnetic field. Also, in both sets of data the characteristic curves obtained for a reference BSA solution having the lowest concentration of 1 mg/mL are presented. In Fig.5.3(a) we see that the only indication for the existence of free BSA in the supernatant of Cs that were prepared at a BSA content of 1 and 2 mg/mL comes from the absorption that emerges below 260 nm. When the preparation of the Cs takes place at a host solution having BSA concentration of 5 mg/mL, a weak distinct absorption at 280 nm shows up owing to free BSA in the supernatant. However, a clear signature of the characteristic absorption at 280 nm evolves only at an even higher BSA content of 6 mg/mL. Figure 5.3(b) presents the respective CD data for the same samples shown in Fig.5.3(a). Even for the lowest BSA concentrations of the host solution, 1 and 2 mg/mL, the CD data reveal some weak indications for the existence of free BSA in the supernatant. When the preparation of the Cs takes place at higher BSA content of the host solution, i.e. 5 and 6 mg/mL, the CD technique provides clear proof of the existence of free BSA in the supernatant; the double peaks that are observed at 208 and 222 nm are characteristic of the α-helical structure. Thus, we can conclude that when the preparation of the Cs takes place at a high BSA content of the host solution, a part of the dissolved BSA does not react with the formed FNs and remains in the supernatant. However, this is only a very small part of the former BSA content as this is clearly proven by the comparison with the CD curve obtained in a reference BSA solution of 1 mg/mL concentration. We stress that the respective curve is multiplied by a factor of $1/14$ in order to be presented in the same scale. It becomes clear that even for a relatively high BSA content of the host solution, i.e. 5 and 6 mg/mL, the dissolved BSA strongly interacts with the formed FNs and is adsorbed onto their surface so that FN-BSA Cs are eventually formed. This is the only explanation for the strong reduction that is observed in the respective CD curves when compared with the one obtained for the reference BSA solution having the modest concentration of 1 mg/mL.

Obviously, both the BSA capacity of FNs and the magnetic properties of the formed FN-BSA Cs are affected by a number of parameters such as the temperature where the reaction is performed and by the BSA concentration of the host solution. These issues are discussed to some extent here since they determine both the biocompatibility/solubility of the produced Cs and the efficiency of their magnetic retraction, which are both key factors for the purposes of the MAHD concept. For this detailed investigation we preferred to use the CD spectropolarimetry technique owing to its superiority on UV-VIS spectrophotometry.

Figures 5.4(a)-5.4(d), 5.5(a)-5.5(d) and 5.6(a)-5.6(d) show CD results for preparations of Cs that were performed under mild stirring at $T_{reac} = 25\ ^oC$, $T_{reac} = 2\ ^oC$, and $T_{reac} = 40\ ^oC$, respectively, for constant FNs content and various BSA concentrations. Open circles refer to supernatant samples after the Fe_3O_4-BSA Cs have been trapped by means of an external magnetic field. Solid circles refer to samples that were obtained after adequate stirring. Finally, circles with crosses refer to reference BSA solutions having the respective concentration. We clearly see that in almost all cases the supernatant samples exhibit lower Θ values when compared to the stirred ones. This clearly proves that the effective BSA concentration is higher in the stirred samples owing to the binding of BSA molecules with the Fe_3O_4 FNs. The temperature where the FN-BSA Cs preparation takes place strongly

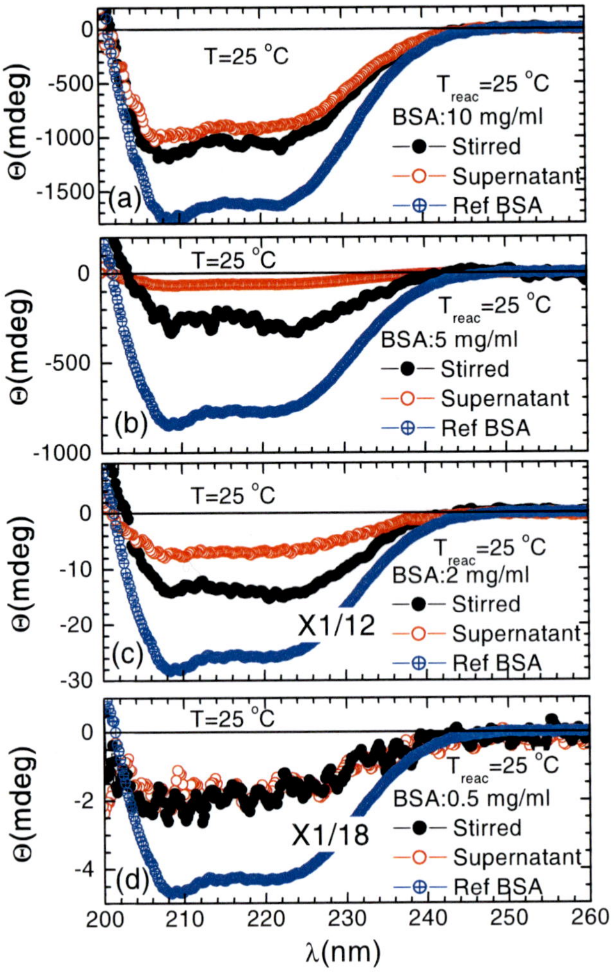

Figure 5.4. CD data for Fe_3O_4-BSA Cs that were prepared at $T_{reac} = 25\ ^oC$. The FNs content is constant, while the BSA concentration varies: 10 mg/mL (a), 5 mg/mL (b), 2 mg/mL (c), and 0.5 mg/mL (d). Open circles refer to supernatant samples after the Fe_3O_4-BSA Cs have been retracted by means of an external magnetic field, while solid circles refer to samples that were obtained after mild stirring. Circles with crosses refer to the respective reference BSA solutions. All measurements were performed at $T = 25\ ^oC$ [Reproduced from Ref. [34]]

influences the CD data. We see that at $T_{reac} = 2\ ^oC$ the difference in the CD data that are obtained in supernatant and stirred samples is more pronounced when compared to the respective ones for the Cs produced at $T_{reac} = 25\ ^oC$. This proves that the conjugation is more successful when the preparation is performed at $T_{reac} = 2\ ^oC$. Thus, the biocompatibility/solubility of Cs produced at $T_{reac} = 2\ ^oC$ should be enhanced when compared to the ones that are produced at $T_{reac} = 25\ ^oC$. Interestingly, the experiments that were performed at $T_{reac} = 40\ ^oC$ exhibit both qualitative and quantitative similarities to the ones obtained at $T_{reac} = 2\ ^oC$.

In all cases the signal of the reference BSA sample is higher when compared to the

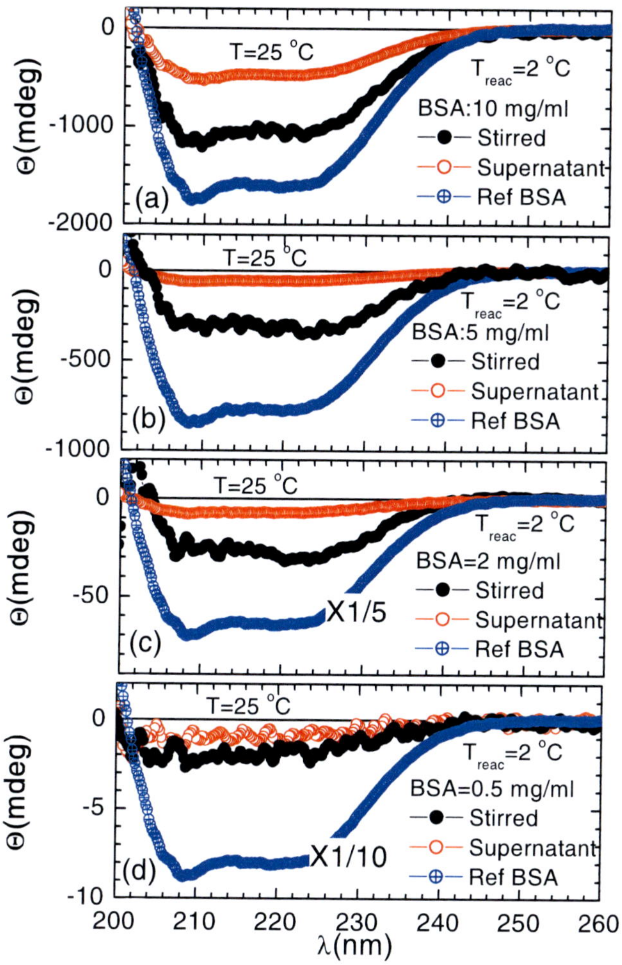

Figure 5.5. CD data for Fe_3O_4-BSA Cs that were prepared at $T_{reac} = 2\ ^oC$. The FNs content is constant, while the BSA concentration varies: 10 mg/mL (a), 5 mg/mL (b), 2 mg/mL (c), and 0.5 mg/mL (d). Open circles refer to supernatant samples after the Fe_3O_4-BSA Cs have been retracted by means of an external magnetic field, while solid circles refer to samples that were obtained after mild stirring. Circles with crosses refer to the respective reference BSA solutions. All measurements were performed at $T = 25\ ^oC$.

respective ones of both the supernatant and stirred samples. Also, we see that especially for the Cs that are prepared in low BSA concentration the relative differences that are observed in the data coming from the supernatant and stirred samples are not so pronounced (see Figs.5.4(d), 5.5(d) and 5.6(d)). At first sight this could be taken as an indication of almost zero surface coverage of the FNs by BSA molecules. However, as it is discussed right below a more thorough analysis of the obtained results that takes into account the specific characteristics of the FN-BSA Cs reveals a more reliable interpretation.

The experimental results presented in Figs. 5.4(a)-5.4(d), 5.5(a)-5.5(d) and 5.6(a)-5.6(d) can be consistently explained as follows: the Fe_3O_4 FNs have a rather big size so

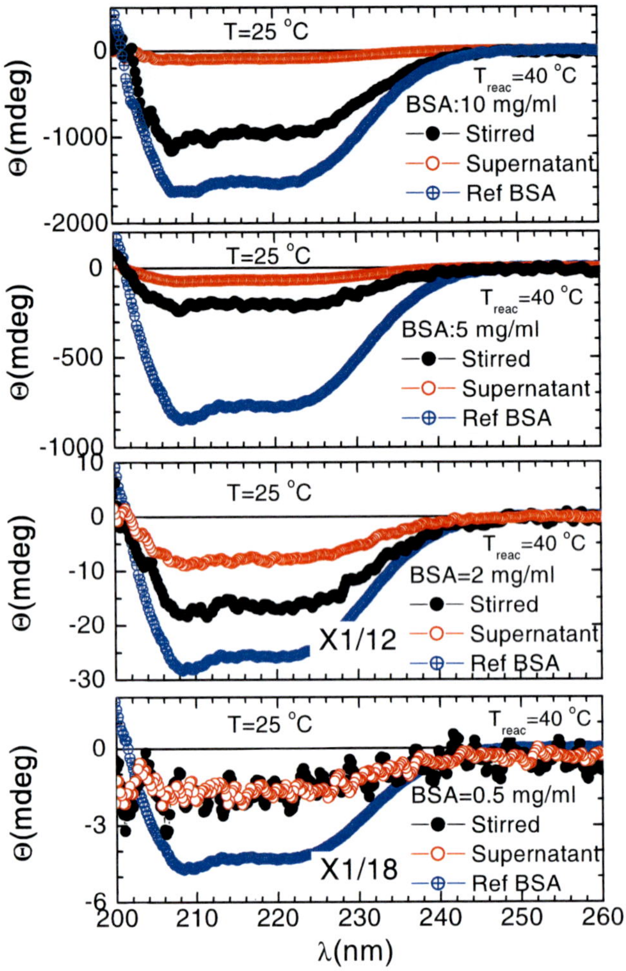

Figure 5.6. CD data for Fe_3O_4-BSA Cs that were prepared at $T_{reac} = 40\ ^oC$. The FNs content is constant, while the BSA concentration varies: 10 mg/mL (a), 5 mg/mL (b), 2 mg/mL (c), and 0.5 mg/mL (d). Open circles refer to supernatant samples after the Fe_3O_4-BSA Cs have been retracted by means of an external magnetic field, while solid circles refer to samples that were obtained after mild stirring. Circles with crosses refer to the respective reference BSA solutions. All measurements were performed at $T = 25\ ^oC$.

that since they are not transparent, during the CD experiments the incident polarized-light beam experiences strong scattering. Consequently, the BSA molecules that are adsorbed onto the FNs are effectively obscured owing to their much smaller size in comparison to their host carriers. Obviously, owing to the decrease of the relative cross-section, also the effective BSA concentration will be apparently reduced in the stirred samples. Thus, we expect that the underlying relative difference in the BSA concentration between the supernatant and stirred samples should be much more pronounced in reality. This specific topic is modelled and discussed in detail elsewhere. [44]

To clearly prove the fact that the BSA concentration of the host solution determines the

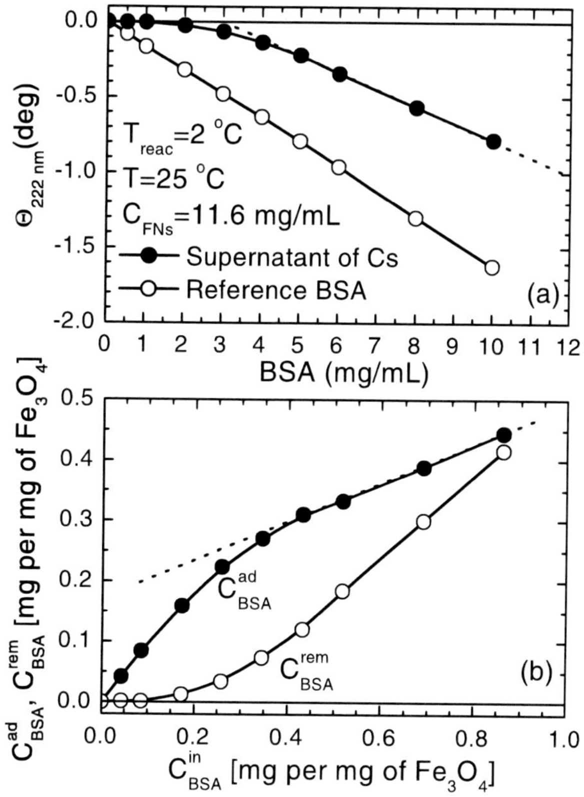

Figure 5.7. (a) Θ values recorded at constant $\lambda = 222$ nm obtained in supernatants of Cs that were produced at $T_{reac} = 2\ ^{o}C$ under systematic variation of the BSA concentration (solid circles), along with the respective reference BSA solutions (open circles), on the initial BSA concentration. In these Cs the nominal concentration of FNs was $C_{FNs} = 11.6$ mg/mL. (b) The estimated BSA concentration that remains in the supernatant (open circles) and adsorbed onto the FNs (solid circles) [normalized per mg of Fe_3O_4]. The measurements were performed at T= 25 ^{o}C.

BSA content of the formed FN-BSA Cs, in Figs.5.7(a)-5.7(b) we present CD data obtained on the supernatant of different Cs that were produced under mild stirring at $T_{reac} = 2\ ^{o}C$. These data were compared with the respective ones obtained for reference BSA solutions. Figure 5.7(a) presents CD results obtained on the supernatant of Cs prepared under different BSA concentration. These CD data refer to the variation of the specific Θ value at $\lambda = 222$ nm, that is characteristic of the a-helical structure of BSA, upon the systematic variation of the BSA concentration. In these Cs the nominal concentration of FNs was $C_{FNs} = 11.6$ mg/mL. We clearly see that for Cs prepared at low BSA concentrations the CD signal of the supernatant is almost zero. This indicates that in these samples all the BSA of the host solution has been adsorbed onto FNs. In contrast, above a threshold BSA concentration (approximately 2 mg/mL) the recorded Θ values exhibit a smooth increase that evolves to a linear variation suggesting that the coverage of FNs tends to saturate so that BSA is not farther drastically adsorbed onto them. Figure 5.7(b) presents the conjugation capacity of the FNs for BSA as was estimated from the raw CD data.

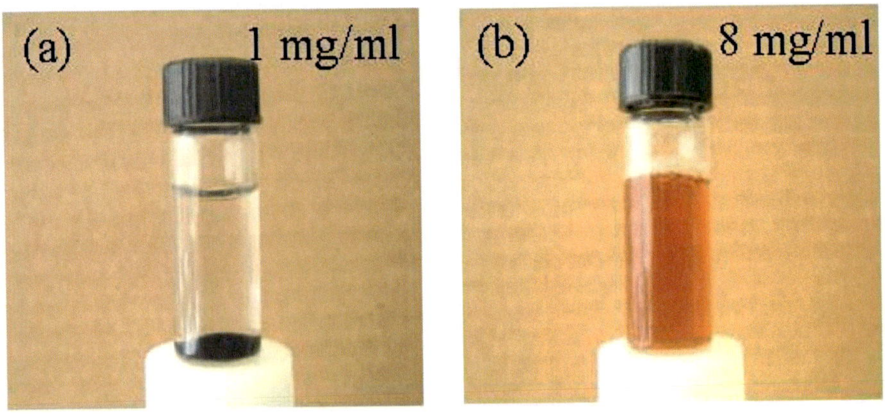

Figure 5.8. (a) Cs prepared under low BSA concentration of the host solution (1 mg/mL) are not saline soluble since they precipitate in a few minutes. (b) In contrast, the ones that are produced in a rich BSA environment (8 mg/mL) are perfectly saline soluble, since they do not precipitate in months duration. [34]

As discussed above, a higher BSA concentration of the host solution results in higher surface coverage of the produced FNs. This will surely improve both the biocompatibility and solubility of the produced FN-TBS Cs, and also could possibly promote their binding capacity with the TTSs. Indeed, we observed that Cs that are produced under low BSA concentration are not saline soluble since they precipitate in a few minutes, as it is shown in Fig.5.8(a) for a sample produced in a BSA concentration of 1 mg/mL. Cs that are produced under high BSA concentration are perfectly saline soluble as it is presented in Fig.5.8(b) for a sample produced in a BSA concentration of 8 mg/mL. It should be noted that these two samples refer to the two limit cases of very low and very high BSA surface coverage (see Fig.5.7).

The data presented until now prove that the BSA concentration of the host solution clearly determines the solubility of the formed Fe_3O_4-BSA Cs by apparently regulating their surface coverage. It should be noted that the BSA molecules are negatively charged. Thus, we can rightfully conclude that Fe_3O_4-BSA Cs that are produced in low BSA concentration have low surface coverage and exhibit a relatively big size so that attractive magnetostatic dipole interactions of the core FNs prevail over the repulsive electrostatic ones of the shell BSA molecules. Thus, agglomeration of the formed Cs naturally intervenes and eventually their precipitation supervenes under the gravitational force as is observed in Fig.5.8(a). In contrast, Fe_3O_4-BSA Cs that are produced under high BSA content should have high surface coverage and exhibit a small size so that attractive magnetostatic dipole interactions of the core FNs are not significant. Since now the repulsive electrostatic forces of the shell BSA molecules take over, agglomeration and subsequent precipitation of the formed Cs is avoided so that the colloidal behavior observed in Fig.5.8(b) can be successfully attained.

Further investigations on this specific issue were performed by means of XRD experiments. Representative XRD data are shown in Figs.5.9(a)-5.9(b) for Cs prepared in the

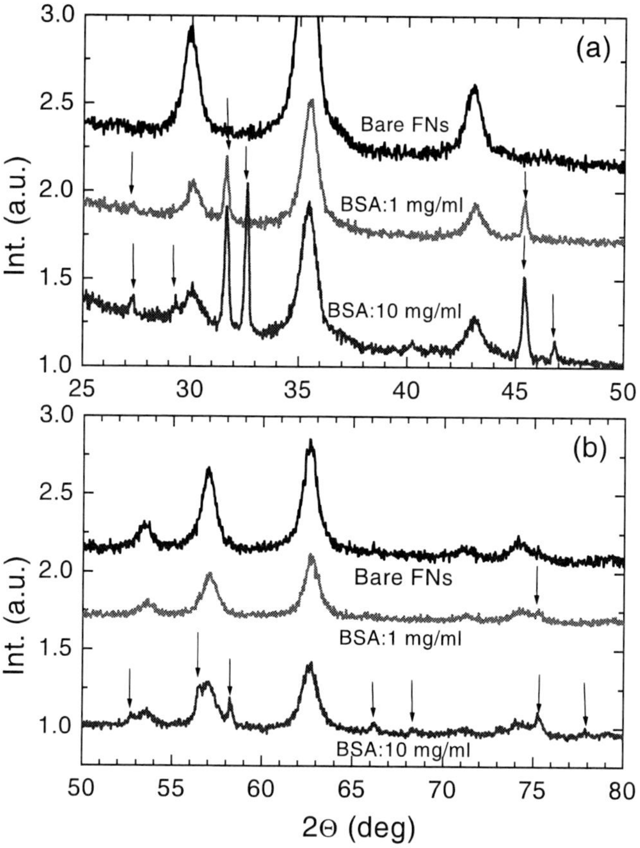

Figure 5.9. Representative XRD data in the range (a) $25^o < 2\Theta < 50^o$ and (b) $50^o < 2\Theta < 80^o$ for the Fe_3O_4-BSA Cs produced under low, 1 mg/mL and high, 10 mg/mL BSA content of the host solution. Careful preparation of the samples to participate in these XRD experiments was followed so that the information of the BSA molecules that were adsorbed on the FNs host carriers to be isolated (see text for details). For the sake of comparison the respective XRD data for bare Fe_3O_4 FNs are also presented.

two limits of very low (1 mg/mL) and very high (10 mg/mL) BSA concentration. We stress that these XRD experiments exclusively refer to Fe_3O_4-BSA Cs that were collected after the original samples had been washed for several times so that free BSA was completely removed. Notice that while free BSA does not exist in the supernatant of the Cs that were prepared in low BSA concentration, in ones that were prepared in high BSA concentration a noticeable amount of free BSA exists. In our XRD experiments we wanted to exclude the contribution of free BSA existing in the supernatant so that the information coming exclusively from the BSA molecules that are adsorbed on the FNs host carriers to be isolated. Careful washing of the former samples guaranties this demand. Especially for the colloid Fe_3O_4-BSA Cs that were prepared under high BSA content we stress that the samples for the XRD experiments were collected from the washed ones after adequate centrifugation at 14000 rpm for 10 min. From the data presented in Figs.5.9(a)-5.9(b) we clearly see that even in the highest BSA concentration of the host solution studied in this book the Fe_3O_4 FNs are formed. However, the height of the diffraction peaks related to the Fe_3O_4 FNs are reduced and some extra peaks emerge as the BSA content increases. These extra peaks can be ascribed to the formation of NH_4-Fe-Cl [Ammonium Iron Chloride] and $(NH_4)4Fe_2(OH)4(CO_3)3 \cdot 3H_2O$ [Ammonium Iron Carbonate Hydroxide Hydrate]. However, they also could be ascribed to Fe_2O_3 [Iron Oxide], $Fe_2O_3 \cdot H_2O$ [Iron Oxide Hydrate], $Fe(OH)_2$ [Iron Hydroxide] and FeO(OH) [Iron Oxide Hydroxide]. We believe that the most plausible scenario relates to the formation of iron complexes having the general form $(NH_4)nFe_m(OH)n(Y) \cdot lH_2O$ owing to the high reactivity of iron with $(NH_4)(OH)$ in aqueous NH_3 solution. Another hint pointing to the validation of this scenario comes from the fact that the formation of these complexes is highly promoted by the presence of BSA; we can assume that since the BSA molecules that are adsorbed on the FNs are negatively charged, they can act as sites where the nucleation of NH_4^+ is motivated under purely electrostatic forces.

Since the formation of the Fe_3O_4-BSA Cs has been proven, the next step for their evaluation refers to their magnetic characterization. Apart from the solubility of the produced Cs, also their magnetic properties are also strongly influenced by their BSA content. We observed that Cs that are produced under low BSA concentration retain the strong magnetic susceptibility of bare FNs, while the ones that are produced in high BSA concentration exhibit suppressed magnetic susceptibility. Detailed measurements were performed by means of a SQUID magnetometer for the magnetic evaluation of the produced Cs. Representative results that were obtained at $T = 40\ ^oC$, $T = 25\ ^oC$, and $T = 2\ ^oC$ are shown in Figs.5.10(a)-5.10(c), respectively for the same Cs for which the CD results were presented in Figs.5.4,5.5 and 5.6. We see that the effective saturation magnetization of the FNs depends on the BSA concentration of the host solution. More specifically, the higher the BSA concentration of the host environment where the preparation of the FNs takes place, the lower the saturation magnetization of the formed Cs. As shown in the following subsection where the magnetic retraction efficiency of the FN-BSA Cs is presented, this fact sets a limit on the magnetic manipulation of these Cs. In order to be appropriate for the MAHD application the Fe_3O_4 FNs should preserve a relatively strong magnetic susceptibility when participating in the Cs, so that generally Cs prepared under relatively low BSA concentration should be preferred. However, low surface coverage of the FNs (Fe_3O_4) with the TBS (BSA) will result in Cs of relatively lower biocompatibility and solubility. Probably for these Cs the binding affinity and capacity with the TTSs will also be reduced. These are serious drawbacks for *in vivo* applications so that for these purposes generally Cs having high BSA content should be preferred and the lower saturation magnetization that they exhibit could be disregarded. These conflicts should be carefully evaluated.

As it becomes clear from the CD and magnetization results that were presented until now, apart from the BSA content of the host solution, the temperature at which the preparation takes place also affects the BSA content and magnetic properties of the formed FN-BSA Cs. In Fig. 5.11 we present the influence of the reaction temperature, T_{reac} on the relative reduction of the formed Cs saturation magnetization when the BSA concentration of the host solution varies by the same amount in all cases. Interestingly, we see that the highest variation of the Cs saturation magnetization is observed when the reaction takes place at temperature $T_{reac} = 25\ ^oC$. In contrast, when the preparation of the Cs takes place

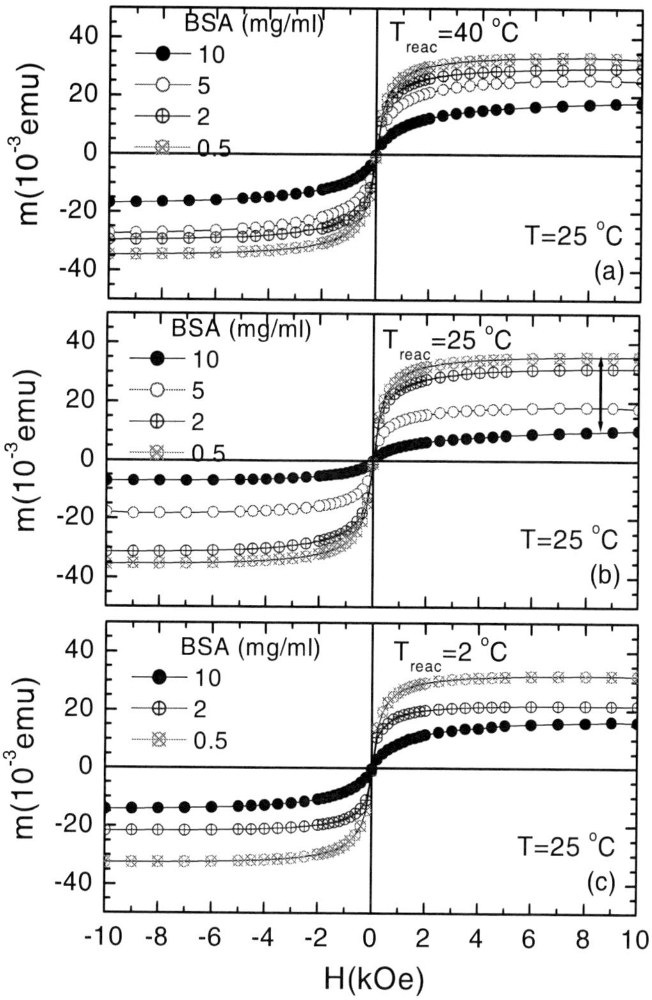

Figure 5.10. Magnetization data for Fe_3O_4-BSA Cs that were prepared at (a) $T_{reac} = 40$ ^oC, (b) $T_{reac} = 25$ ^oC and (c) $T_{reac} = 2$ ^oC. The FNs content is constant, while the BSA concentration varies. The saturation magnetization of the produced FN-BSA Cs depends strongly on their BSA content. All measurements were performed at $T = 25$ ^oC.

at low ($T_{reac} = 2$ ^oC) or relatively higher ($T_{reac} = 55$ ^oC) temperatures, the variation of the saturation magnetization upon the BSA content is significantly lower.

These experimental results suggest that magnetization measurements could be used as an efficient technique for the determination of the BSA concentration of a host solution where the preparation of the FNs takes place. For instance, from the magnetization data shown in Fig.5.11 we can estimate the detection sensitivity for the BSA concentration of a host solution when compared with a standard solution of known BSA concentration. Assuming a 10^{-6} emu sensitivity of a commercial SQUID magnetometer we can obtain a 10^{-6} emu[Δ_{BSA}(mg/mL)/Δm(emu)] detection limit for the BSA concentration by taking into account the variation of the saturation magnetization of the formed Cs (see double arrow in Fig.5.10 (b)) against the variation of the BSA concentration. The respective data are pre-

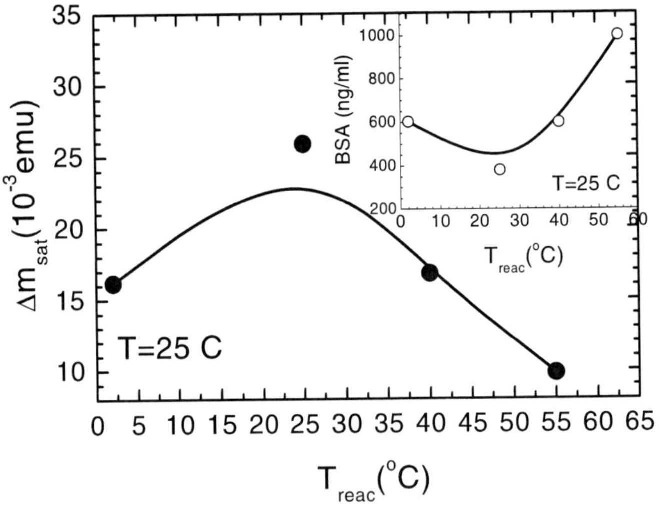

Figure 5.11. Variation of the saturation magnetization of the formed Fe_3O_4-BSA Cs upon variation of the BSA concentration of the host solution for different reaction temperatures, T_{reac} where the preparation took place. The inset presents the BSA concentration that can be detected owing to the variation of the saturation magnetization of the produced Fe_3O_4-BSA Cs. All the values were calculated from magnetization data as the ones presented in Fig.5.10, for Cs that were prepared under mild stirring at $T_{reac} = 2\ ^oC$, 25 ^oC, 40 ^oC and 55 ^oC. In all cases the variation of the BSA content of the host solution where the preparation of the Cs takes place is the same, ranging from 0.5 to 10 mg/mL. All magnetization measurements were performed at T= 25 ^oC.

sented in the inset of Fig.5.11 and refer to samples that were prepared at the same reaction temperatures, T_{reac} shown in the main panel. We see that the calculated values are in the range of ng/mL with the lowest one (380 ng/mL) obtained when the preparation takes place at $T_{reac} = 25\ ^oC$. This value sets the detection limit for the BSA concentration and compares nicely with the one given in Ref. [55], where relative FNs were employed for the detection of extremely low values of human C-reactive protein.

2. In vitro Evaluation of the FN-BSA Cs

The issues discussed above should be carefully evaluated for future *in vivo* applications. The prerequisite of intense magnetic susceptibility (so that easy magnetic retraction can be achieved by means of a "magnetic dialyser") that is observed for Fe_3O_4-BSA Cs of low BSA content should be counterbalanced by the need of biocompatibility/solubility (so that both free circulation and minimum conflict with the immune system can be achieved) that is observed for Cs of high BSA content.

In our *in vitro* experiments we have employed Cs that have both low and high BSA content. First, we will discuss the retraction efficiency of the simple FN-BSA Cs under the application of a magnetic field. Second, the binding affinity and capacity of these Cs with specific TTSs is also discussed in detail.

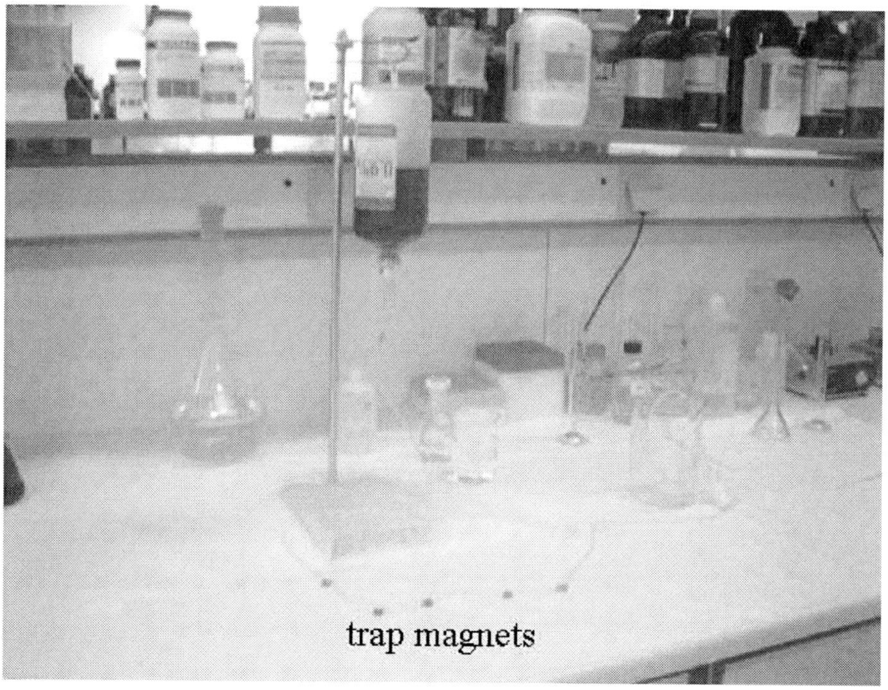

Figure 5.12. (a) Simple experimental set up that is used in the laboratory for the *in vitro* evaluation of the magnetic retraction efficiency and the toxin binding efficiency of the prepared Fe_3O_4-BSA Cs. In these preliminary experiments the concentration of Cs is 0.1 mg/mL, their flow is maintained under gravity and is controlled by a simple flow regulator in the range of 50 – 100 mL/min. Five trap magnets that provide intense field gradients are placed along the circulation line (see Fig.5.13 for details).

2.1. Magnetic Retraction Efficiency of Bare FNs and FN-BSA Cs

The evaluation procedure for this test experiment is as follows: [34] in saline we added Fe_3O_4-BSA Cs at a relatively high concentration of 100 mg/L and we performed sequential circulations under gravity at a flow rate of 50 – 100 mL/min as it is shown in Fig.5.12. For the realization of a simple "magnetic dialyser" (*vide infra*) we placed three to five disc-shape permanent magnets (5 – 10 mm in diameter) along the circulation line. These magnets produce intense magnetic field gradients that are needed for the retraction of Fe_3O_4-BSA Cs; we recall that a homogeneous magnetic field **B** exerts only torque $\mathbf{N}=\mathbf{m}\times\mathbf{B}$ on a FN that can be represented as a point magnetic dipole **m**, but cannot be used for its immobilization since only a magnetic field gradient can immobilize it by exerting a force $\mathbf{F}=\nabla(\mathbf{m}\circ\mathbf{B})$. [109] The maximum magnetic field that these permanent magnets produce, as was measured by means of a Hall sensor, is in the range of 1000 – 1500 Oe. As was expected, the obtained results clearly show that Cs having low BSA content are retracted much more easily than the respective ones of high BSA content. In Figs.5.13(a)-5.13(c) we focus on the trap magnets prior and after the first circulation is completed, respectively, for Cs that were prepared under rigorous vortex stirring at a BSA concentration of 1 mg/mL of the host solution. We observed that the intense magnetic field gradients that are produced at the edges of these disc-shape magnets act as strong magnetic traps for these highly magnetic Cs. This can be clearly resolved in Fig.5.13(c). We also observed that for the highly magnetic Cs their concentration decreases sharply from circulation to circulation, while for the weakly magnetic Cs many more circulations are needed in order for their concentration to be lowered significantly.

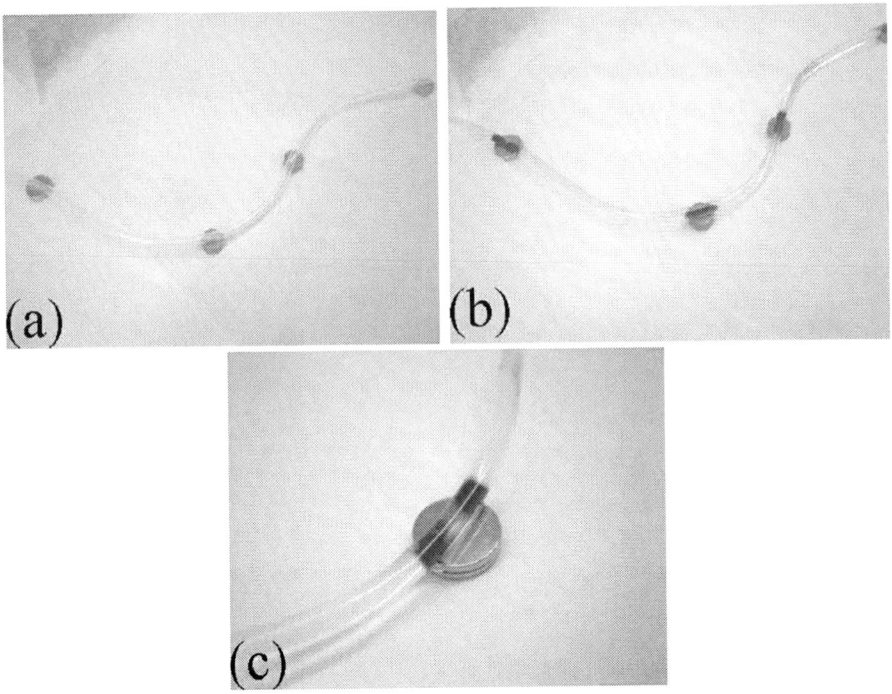

Figure 5.13. Detail of the trap magnets used to retract the FN-BSA Cs that flow at a rate of 50 – 100 mL/min along the circulation line: (a) before, and (b) after the first circulation is completed. (c) Detail of a single trap magnet; intense magnetic field gradients immobilize the FNs mainly at the edges of the magnet.

To quantify these observations we have performed magnetization measurements for samples drawn after each circulation was completed. Figure 5.14 shows the percentage variation of the magnetically estimated concentration of highly magnetic Fe_3O_4-BSA Cs prepared at a BSA concentration of 1 mg/mL at the end of the first four circulations. These data reveal that highly magnetic Fe_3O_4-BSA Cs are entirely retracted after a few circulations.

In contrast to the highly magnetic Cs, in the case of Cs that were prepared in high BSA concentrations (for instance, 10 mg/mL) many more circulations, exceeding 15 – 20, are needed so that a significant amount of them to be retracted (results not shown). Thus, so far as the magnetic retraction efficiency is considered, the Cs prepared under low BSA concentration are ideal. However, as it was discussed above the low BSA content of these Cs makes them poor candidates for *in vivo* applications. Their solubility, and subsequently their biocompatibility, are substandard when compared to the Cs having high BSA surface coverage. Their binding affinity and capacity with TTSs can be reduced as well. Further *in vitro* experiments are surely needed for the detailed evaluation of these

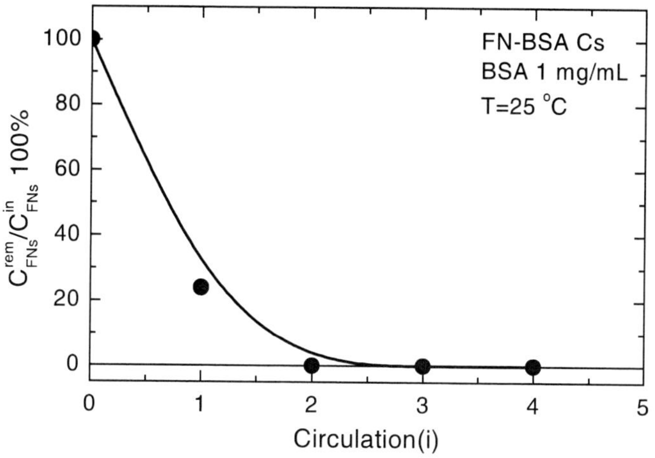

Figure 5.14. Percentage variation of the magnetically estimated remaining concentration of Cs for samples that were drawn at the end of each circulation. The data refer to highly magnetic Cs that were prepared at a low BSA concentration of 1 mg/mL. The initial concentration of FNs was $C_{FNs} = 100$ mg/L. The measurements were performed at T$= 25\ ^{o}$C.

conflicting issues so that the most appropriate candidate Cs are employed in future *in vivo* applications. *According to our investigations, probably the most appropriate Cs for the utilization of the MAHD concept are these produced at a BSA concentration of about* 2 – 6 *mg/mL (see Fig.5.7) since in these Cs the FNs have the maximum BSA surface coverage and are still highly magnetic. Thus, in these Cs the prerequisites of biocompatibility, solubility and high magnetic retraction efficiency are met equally well.*

2.2. Toxin Binding Affinity and Capacity of Bare FNs and FN-BSA Cs

In order to demonstrate the *in vitro* applicability of the MAHD method in this subsection we present results on the toxin binding affinity and capacity of both bare FNs and FN-BSA Cs. Three toxins, namely homocysteine, p-Cresol and β2-microglobulin served as model TTSs in these *in vitro* experiments. These specific toxins were selected for two basic reasons: first, they have an important biological impact not only for the ESRD patients on HD therapy but also for the general population (see the discussion made below), and second, owing to their protein binding affinity despite their small (homocysteine and p-cresol) or middle (β2-microglobulin) MW they form large conjugate molecules that are not efficiently removed with the semipermeable membranes that are used in conventional HD.

We stress that all the presented results refer to the case where after their preparation both bare FNs and FN-BSA Cs were adequately washed by commercially available sodium chloride 0.9% w/v. This process removed any excessive NH_4OH so that final redispersion in sodium chloride 0.9% w/v yields a suspension/solution (depending on the BSA surface coverage as discussed above) that has the neutral pH$= 6.5$ of pure saline (notice that right after preparation pH$= 9 - 9.5$ due to excessive NH_4OH; see subsection VI.B "Preparation of samples"). This process is definitely needed in order to clearly show that the prepared bare FNs and FN-BSA Cs are able to bind with the target toxins under physiological pH conditions that are met in *in vivo* applications.

2.2.1. Homocysteine

First we discuss these topics for homocysteine (Hcy) that is a toxin of great biological importance having the formula $HSCH_2CH_2CH(NH_2)CO_2H$, MW= 135 D and the respective structure that is schematically shown in Fig.5.15(a). Hcy is an intermediary substance evolving during the metabolism of the sulfur-containing amino acid methionine. Especially, since it is formed from methionine it can be either remethylated under the action of B_{12}-dependent methionine synthase so that methionine is recovered, or transformed to cysteine (Cys) following an alternative B_6-dependent biochemical pathway. Since both processes strongly depend on the existence of basic B vitamins, including folate, cyanocobalamin (B_{12}), and pyridoxine hydrochloride (B_6) increased blood levels of Hcy can serve as a marker of vitamin B deficiency or inadequate processing.

Owing to the existence of the functional thiol group -S-H (or sulfhydryl group) Hcy exhibits intense biochemical action. Thus, in human plasma Hcy can be seen in both reduced and oxidized forms. Hcy refers only to the reduced form (or sulfhydryl form) where the hydrogen atom of the thiol group is preserved, while the oxidized form (or disulfide form) refers to the case where the hydrogen atoms are rejected under the formation of a favorable -S-S- covalent bond which is called a disulfide bond. Hcy participates in such bonds (i) with another Hcy molecule resulting in the dimer Hcy-S-S-Hcy (called homocystine) as it is schematically shown in Fig.5.15(b), (ii) with a Cys candidate in the form Hcy-S-S-Cys as it is schematically shown in Fig.5.15(c), and (iii) with proteins that contain susceptible Cys residues so that a complex protein-Cys-S-S-Hcy is constructed as it is schematically shown in Fig.5.15(d). The latter structure hosts most of the Hcy existing in blood serum (approximately $80-90\%$), while the rest Hcy content of blood serum resides to the other two forms, Hcy-S-S-Hcy and Hcy-S-S-Cys in almost equal amounts (approximately $5-10\%$ each). Finally, referring to the reduced form of Hcy, it exists in blood serum in only minor amounts (approximately 1%). When referring to the total Hcy (tHcy) existing in human plasma we take into account both the reduced and various oxidized forms of Hcy. In contrast, the free Hcy (fHcy) fraction refers only to the reduced form of Hcy.

Nowadays, it is accepted that tHcy has an important biological impact since even mild hyperhomocysteinemia are associated with premature atherosclerosis, [110–112] CVD, [113–118] memory deficit, [119] and with Alzheimer's disease. [120,121] The normal and pathological blood levels can be seen in Table 5.1. A compact review on these topics can be found in Ref. [23]. Especially for the ESRD patients on HD therapy, it is well known that elevated blood levels of tHcy are associated with thrombotic episodes. [24] For these patients sufficient vascular access and stable hemodynamic status are of great importance for the maintenance of an adequate HD dose. Thus, the selective removal of substances such as Hcy that play a major role in thrombotic episodes that could deteriorate the vascular network of the forearm where the arteriovenous fistula is hosted could be of great importance for ESRD patients.

Whether increased tHcy plasma level is causal, so that it could be considered as an independent risk factor, or merely an event so that could act as a simple marker for CVD

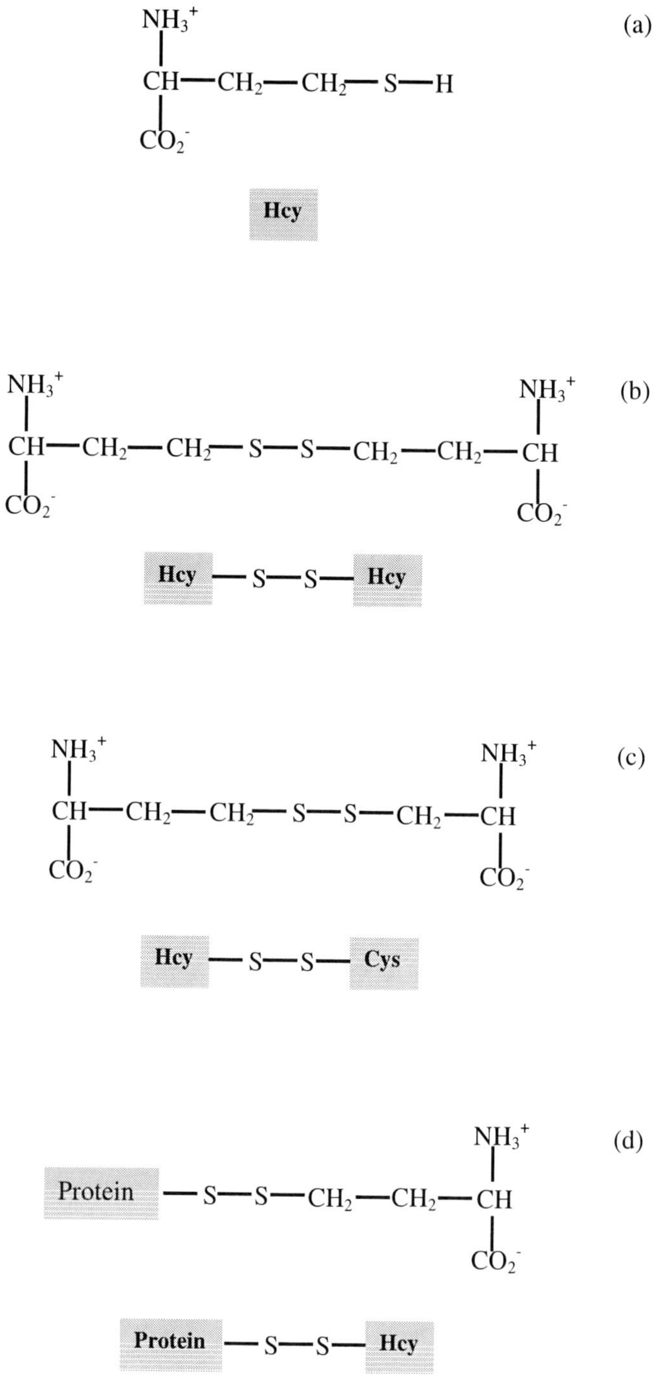

Figure 5.15. Schematic illustrations of the structure of (a) reduced Hcy and of its various oxidized forms originating by disulfide bonds with (b) another Hcy molecule, (c) a Cys molecule, and (d) a protein.

Table 5.1. Normal and pathological tHcy blood levels. [116]

Condition	tHcy (μmol/L)
Normal	5-15
Mild	15-25
Intermediate	25-50
Severe	50-500

and related diseases, is still under investigation not only for the ESRD patients but also for the general population. [23–25] However, two recent studies have provided strong indications (if not proofs) that indeed increased tHcy is causal for CVD. First, F. Pizzolo et al. reported a study on 180 patients having coronary artery disease and impaired renal function (GFR ranging in 67 – 79 mL/min/1.73 m^2). [26] This study [26] provided evidence that tHcy could be considered as a risk factor since the authors reported that *as the levels of tHcy increase, a lower number of traditional risk factors is needed so that the same degree of coronary atherosclerosis to be observed.* Second, M. Suliman et al. reported a careful analysis of results that were obtained on 317 patients during a 66 months follow-up. [27] This study [27] revealed that although a first evaluation of the data implied that increased tHcy levels were not associated with CVD, *a reanalysis that takes into account additional parameters, including the overall nutritional and inflammation status, restores the expectation that increased tHcy concentration is related to increased CVD and mortality.* We believe that these two recent studies [26,27] provide evidence that tHcy could be definitely considered as an independent risk factor for CVD. This is why we have chosen Hcy as one of the significant TTSs studied in our work.

Whether tHcy is a primary causal factor that massively motivates the various diseases mentioned above or has a secondary role through exerting a synergetic effect along with other well-established risk factors (such as HT, DM, HC, smoking, vascular calcification etc), owing to its overall biological significance it is well accepted that even slightly elevated blood levels should be restored to the normal values. Especially for high-risk groups such as CVD and ESRD patients extra provision should be taken. Thus, first-line lowering strategies of tHcy rely on supplementation of folate, B_{12}, and B_6 vitamins. [113–116] Other Hcy lowering strategies based on supplementation of betaine, serine, creatine and dialysis with high-flux filters have also been employed. [122] However, many cases of not only severe hyperhomocysteinemia but also of mild hyperhomocysteinemia (see Table 5.1) cannot be handled adequately by neither of these techniques so that Hcy levels remain above normal in a significant patients population. [114–116, 122–124]

Generally, Hcy was selected for demonstrating the *in vitro* applicability of MAHD for two basic reasons: First, its significant biological impact for the ESRD patients. Second, the inability of conventional HD to remove efficiently this toxin owing to its protein binding affinity. Specifically, apart from these two basic reasons Hcy was chosen as a favorable candidate TTS owing to the following technical ones: [34,35]

(i) It is well known that the thiol group -S-H exhibits intense reactivity with transition metals [125,126] so that it is generally expected that even bare Fe_3O_4 FNs could act as TBS for Hcy leading to the formation of complex Fe_3O_4-S-Hcy.

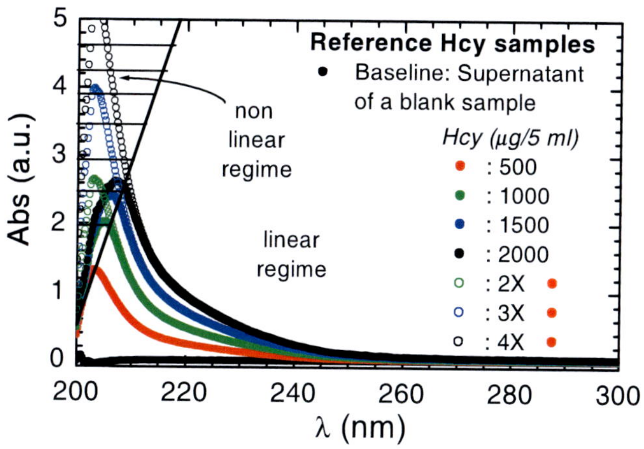

Figure 5.16. UV-VIS absorption data (focused in the range of 200 – 300 nm) for Hcy reference samples at various concentrations 500, 1000, 1500, and 2000 $\mu g/5$ mL. The solid circles represent raw experimental data, while the open circles correspond to the raw data of the 500 $\mu g/5$ mL sample when multiplied by appropriate factors so that the regime where the linear behavior holds to be surveyed.

(ii) The formation of Fe_3O_4-BSA Cs could further promote the binding of Hcy onto these Cs since BSA, similarly to HSA, apart from the 17 intrachain disulfide bonds formed between Cys residues, at site 34 hosts a free Cys residue [127,128] that, although partially protected, is still a promising candidate for binding with Hcy through a disulfide bond. Thus, we expected that the Fe_3O_4-BSA Cs should exhibit higher binding capacity for the Hcy TTS when compared to the bare Fe_3O_4 FNs leading to the formation of Hcy-S-Fe_3O_4-BSA-S-S-Hcy complexes.

(iii) Finally, transition metals react rapidly with Hcy through the chemically active thiol group [129–131] so that it is generally hoped that bare Fe_3O_4 FNs could serve the basic prerequisite of MAHD related to the prompt binding of the FN-TBS Cs with the TTSs at short times right after administration. We have to recall that although the FN-TBS Cs should be administered timely prior to the MAHD session, long residence times cannot be used in order to avoid noticeable interaction with the reticuloendothelial system that would seriously decrease the provision of Cs remaining in the blood stream (for a review of this topic see Ref. [106] and references therein). Unfortunately, for this specific purpose the addition of BSA probably cannot offer any further improvement: as was mentioned above, in both BSA and HSA site 34 hosts a free Cys residue [127, 128] that unfortunately is partially protected since it is placed approximately 10 $\mathring{A}$ deep in a crevice between helices h2 and h3 in subdomain IA. [127,128,132,133] Thus, HSA exhibits relatively slow binding dynamics with Hcy that extend in the range of hours for an important Hcy fraction to bind with HSA. [134] Supposing that the same binding dynamics holds for BSA and Hcy we can conclude that the addition of BSA onto the FNs not only would not improve but would probably degrade the binding dynamics between bare FNs and Hcy. These details should be further elucidated in the near future.

We have performed systematic measurements to resolve the binding affinity and capacity of both bare Fe_3O_4 FNs and Fe_3O_4-BSA Cs for Hcy. Three different techniques were employed in order to quantify our experiments: UV-VIS spectrophotometry, Nuclear Magnetic Resonance (NMR) and the standard Fluorescence Polarization Immunoassay (FPIA) method that is used in clinical practice.

UV-VIS spectrophotometry: Before presenting the UV-VIS results we will briefly justify the applicability of the technique for the estimation of the Hcy concentration. UV-VIS spectrophotometry relates to the absorption of photons in the visible and near ultraviolet range of electromagnetic spectrum by molecules that undergo electronic transitions. The Beer-Lambert law quantifies this process by using a linear dependence between the absorption and the concentration of the solution. Due to its simplicity, the UV-VIS technique is routinely used for the determination of the concentration of a solution. However, before any quantification is made we have to confirm the validity of the linear relation for the range of Hcy concentrations used in our experiments. In Fig.5.16 we present UV-VIS data for four different Hcy concentrations in saline solution. Solid points refer to raw experimental data, while open points refer to the experimental data for the lowest Hcy concentration (500 μg/5 mL) that are multiplied by appropriate factors in order the linearity with the respective experimental curves to be validated. We clearly see that depending on the concentration there is a regime where the linear behavior holds. However, as the Hcy concentration increases the linear behavior is progressively limited to higher wavelengths. Thus, any estimation of the effective Hcy concentration by means of UV-VIS measurements should be limited outside the hatched regime shown in Fig.5.16.

Once the Hcy concentration-absorption linear regime has been surveyed we can use this technique to estimate the adsorption of Hcy onto both bare Fe_3O_4 FNs and Fe_3O_4-BSA Cs. Figures 5.17(a)-5.17(d) present systematic results obtained in the supernatant of Fe_3O_4-BSA Cs having different BSA content (bare Fe_3O_4 FNs refer to zero BSA content). We recall that after their preparation the Fe_3O_4-BSA Cs were washed adequately with saline in order excessive NH_4OH to be removed. Finally, they were redispersed in saline so that the resulted suspension has pH= 6.5. Afterwards, Hcy is added and adequate stirring follows (for a couple of minutes) without any further treatment. Routinely, after waiting for an hour we retract the Fe_3O_4-BSA Cs by means of an externally applied magnetic field and we collect the supernatant. The UV-VIS absorption data obtained for each supernatant provide information for the remaining concentration of Hcy by performing a direct comparison with the relative curve obtained on the respective reference Hcy solution. In this way the exact Hcy amount that is adsorbed onto the Cs may be easily determined. A practical issue of technical interest that should be clearly mentioned here is that in these UV-VIS measurements as baseline we used the supernatant of a Hcy-free Fe_3O_4-BSA Cs sample that it was prepared following the same preparation conditions. Thus, all the curves measured in each series reveal exclusively the remaining concentration of Hcy in the supernatant. In Figs.5.17(a)-5.17(d) we show only two representative reference curves having a Hcy content of 500 μg/5 mL (dotted curve) and 1000 μg/5 mL (dashed curve). From these data we can easily see that after Hcy has reacted with the Fe_3O_4-BSA Cs, the remaining concentration in the supernatant reduces strongly when compared to its initial value. For instance, the curve obtained for an initial Hcy content of 2000 μg/5 mL almost coincides with the reference one having Hcy content 500 μg/5 mL. *Proving our former expectation, these systematic data reveal that Hcy reacts extensively with both the bare Fe_3O_4 FNs*

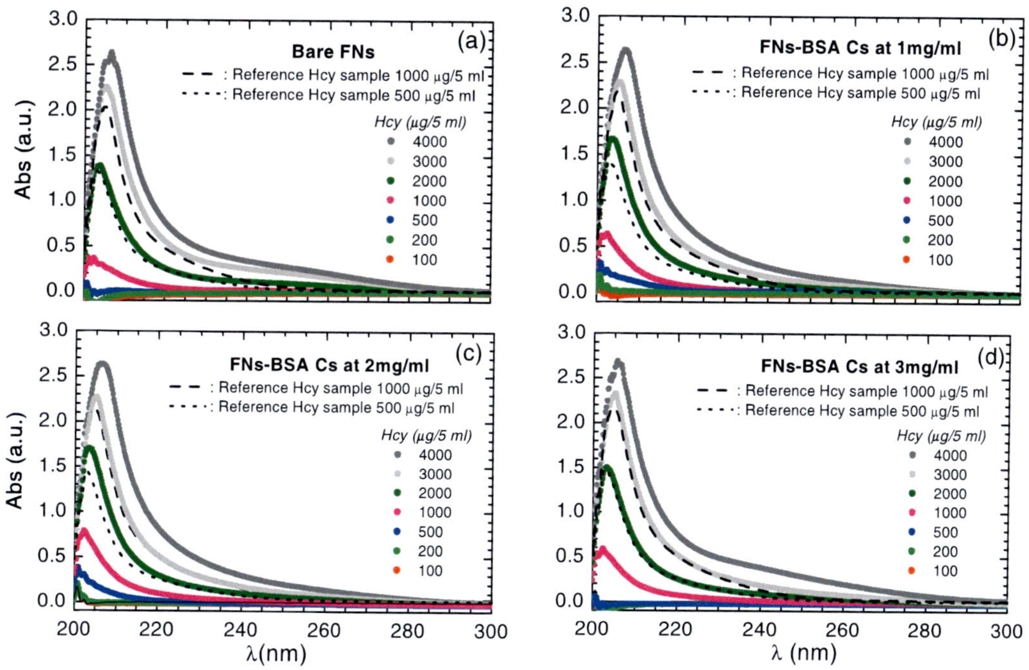

Figure 5.17. UV-VIS absorption data (focused in the range of 200 – 300 nm) for the supernatant of various FN-BSA Cs that were prepared at different BSA content of the host solution, (a) 0 mg/mL (bare FNs), (b) 1 mg/mL, (c) 2 mg/mL, and (d) 3 mg/mL. In all cases, systematically increasing amounts of Hcy were added ranging from 100 to 4000 $\mu g/5$ mL. For the sake of comparison, in all cases two Hcy reference samples having concentrations 500 (dotted curve) and 1000 (dashed curve) $\mu g/5$ mL are shown.

(Fig.5.17(a)) and the Fe_3O_4-BSA Cs (Figs.5.17(b)-5.17(d)). Furthermore, the presence of BSA seems to slightly increase the binding capacity of the Fe_3O_4-BSA Cs with Hcy. These results are quantified and discussed late on when the respective data obtained by NMR and FPIA are presented. However, at this point we should stress that these data reveal the following impressive fact: Hcy content up to 500 $\mu g/5$ mL (740 μmol/L) is completely adsorbed onto the bare Fe_3O_4 and the Fe_3O_4-BSA Cs. This Hcy concentration is far above the limits of severe hyperhomocysteinemia shown in Table 5.1. This means that even severe hyperhomocysteinemia could be treated by means of MAHD. A caution that should be stressed is that the amount of FNs employed in these experiments is extremely high (50 mmol/L). Below we will present results on significantly lower FNs concentrations and we will examine their range of effectiveness in adsorbing Hcy.

At this point the binding dynamics of both bare Fe_3O_4 FNs and Fe_3O_4-BSA Cs with Hcy should be discussed since this issue is related to one basic prerequisite of MAHD. The presence of the FN-TBS Cs in the patient blood stream should only be transient so that noticeable interaction with the reticuloendothelial system to be avoided. Thus, although the FN-TBS Cs should be administered timely prior to the MAHD session (30 – 120 min), long residence times cannot be used; the FN-TBS Cs should exhibit intense binding dynamics with the TTSs so that they will be able to collect them promptly, before the immune system

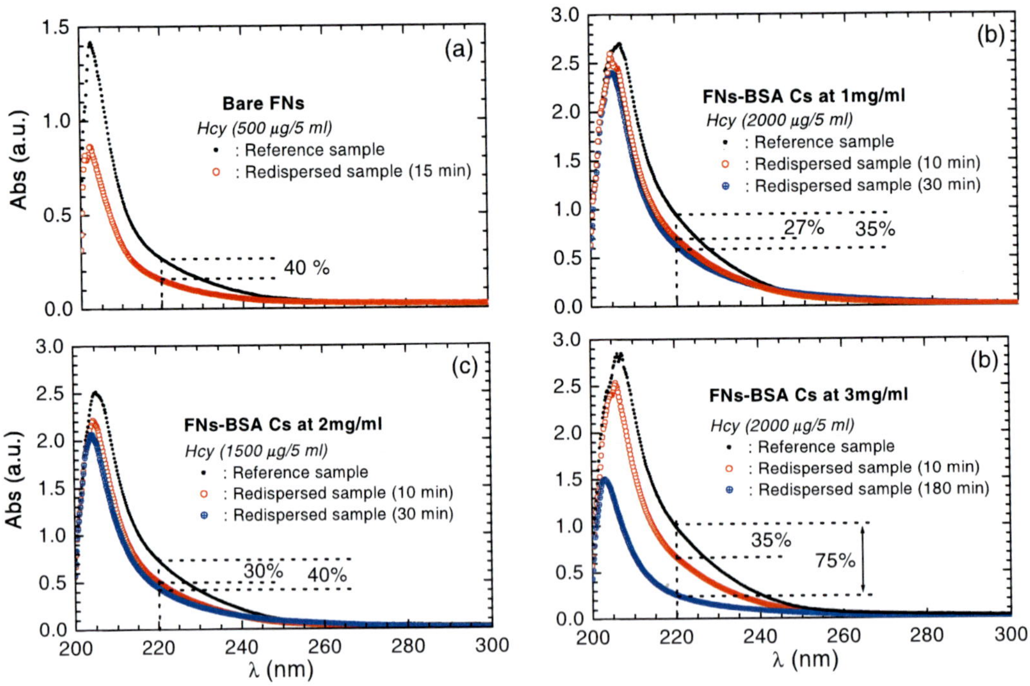

Figure 5.18. UV-VIS absorption data (focused in the range of 200 − 300 nm) revealing the binding dynamics between Fe_3O_4-BSA Cs and Hcy (see text for details). The presented data correspond to Cs prepared at BSA content of (a) 0 mg/mL (bare FNs), (b) 1 mg/mL, (c) 2 mg/mL, and (d) 3 mg/mL. The Hcy content varies for each case.

is triggered. The results shown in Figs.5.18(a)-5.18(d) refer to various Hcy and BSA contents and reveal the time scale over which bare Fe_3O_4 and Fe_3O_4-BSA Cs react with Hcy so that a noticeable Hcy decrease is observed in the supernatant. We note that the set of curves presented in each panel were obtained on a *single* sample according to the following process: initially, a sample of bare Fe_3O_4 or Fe_3O_4-BSA Cs was prepared, the Cs were retracted by an external magnetic field and the supernatant was drawn. At this stage the supernatant was used for obtaining the baseline for the subsequent UV-VIS measurements. After having recorded the baseline, Hcy was added to the supernatant and the respective curve was measured (indicated as reference sample in Figs.5.18(a)-5.18(d)). Subsequently, the bare Fe_3O_4 or Fe_3O_4-BSA Cs were redispersed to the supernatant and adequate stirring followed for a couple of minutes. The suspension was left without any further treatment for a desired time duration and then the bare Fe_3O_4 or Fe_3O_4-BSA Cs were retracted so that the UV-VIS data could be obtained for the supernatant. *Proving our former expectation these systematic data reveal that the binding of Hcy onto both bare Fe_3O_4 and Fe_3O_4-BSA Cs proceeds promptly exhibiting a reduction of* 30 − 45% *within the first* 10 − 15 *min.* This result agrees favorably with the related literature referring to the binding dynamics of Hcy with another transition metal, namely Au nanoparticles. [129–131] Furthermore, it seems that bare Fe_3O_4 exhibit faster binding dynamics when compared to Fe_3O_4-BSA Cs. This is in agreement with the obvious expectation that as the FNs are progressively loaded with BSA the relatively slower dynamics [134] governing the binding between BSA and Hcy should predominate over the comparatively faster processes [129–131] occurring between Fe_3O_4 and Hcy.

Nuclear Magnetic Resonance spectroscopy: Despite the fact that the UV-VIS spectrophotometry has already provided important information for the estimation of the Hcy concentration remaining in the supernatants and the subsequent evaluation of the respective binding capacity of the bare Fe_3O_4 and the Fe_3O_4-BSA Cs, additional information coming from other spectroscopic and biochemical techniques is surely needed in order for these indirect results to be fairly justified.

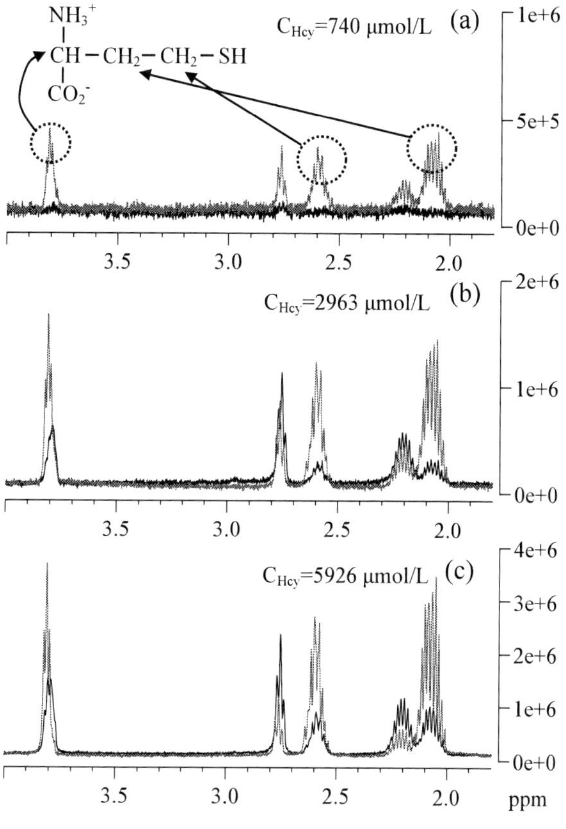

Figure 5.19. Comparative ^{1}H NMR spectra for the determination of the Hcy concentration remaining in the supernatant after its reaction with bare Fe_3O_4 FNs. Black curves correspond to the supernatant drawn from each sample after Hcy has been adsorbed onto the FNs, while grey (red) curves correspond to the respective reference Hcy solutions having the same concentrations of (a) $C_{Hcy} = 740$, (b) 2963, and (c) 5926 μmol/L. In these experiments the FNs concentration was $C_{FNs} = 50$ mmol/L [Reproduced from Ref. [34]].

Thus, we have performed ^{1}H Nuclear Magnetic Resonance (NMR) experiments in the supernatant of the same samples that were studied with UV-VIS spectrophotometry. Representative results are shown in Figs.5.19-5.20 for bare Fe_3O_4 FNs and Fe_3O_4-BSA Cs (BSA= 3 mg/mL), respectively for a FNs concentration of 50 mmol/L. The results shown in both Figs.5.19-5.20 were obtained on supernatants that were typically drawn 4 – 5 hours after Hcy was added to the FNs suspension. In Figs.5.19-5.20 we also present the results coming from the respective Hcy reference samples for a straightforward comparison. The assignment of each resonance observed in the NMR spectrum to the respective ^{1}H nuclei is schematically shown in each case.

From these comparative data the effective adsorption of Hcy onto bare Fe_3O_4 FNs (Fig.5.19) and Fe_3O_4-BSA Cs (Fig.5.20) can be determined. We observe that in both cases a Hcy concentration of $C_{Hcy} = 740$ μmol/L is completely adsorbed onto both bare Fe_3O_4 FNs and Fe_3O_4-BSA Cs so that no Hcy is detected in the supernatant. In contrast, the same Hcy concentration can be easily resolved in a reference sample of the same Hcy concentration. The binding capacity of bare FNs and FN-BSA Cs saturates at a slightly higher Hcy concentration so that ultimately for a concentration of 1481 μmol/L Hcy is clearly observed in the supernatant. Regarding the reduction of the Hcy concentration upon adsorption onto both bare Fe_3O_4 FNs and Fe_3O_4-BSA Cs these ^{1}H NMR data are in complete agreement with the UV-VIS results that were presented above. This will be fully elucidated below, where all the data obtained by the three different techniques, namely UV-VIS spectrophotometry, NMR spectroscopy and FPIA method are comparatively presented.

Figures 5.21-5.22 show comparatively the respective ^{1}H NMR data for the determination of the Hcy concentration in supernatants drawn from the bare Fe_3O_4 (Fig.5.21) and the Fe_3O_4-BSA Cs (Fig.5.22) samples when these are freshly prepared ($4-5$ hours after the addition of Hcy) and after incubation for a minimum of 12 hours. From these data we see that after incubation the resonance peaks originally occurring at 2.07 and 2.58 ppm disappear completely for both the bare Fe_3O_4 and the Fe_3O_4-BSA Cs. Instead, the relative peaks that emerge at 2.20 and 2.77 ppm increase in intensity indicating that the chemical environment of the respective ^{1}H nuclei (see the assignment made in the schematic inset) is drastically altered. We ascribe this strong alteration of the nuclear resonance landscape to the dimer homocystine that is formed via disulfide bonds between the free Hcy molecules existing in the supernatant. Once the dimer homocystine is formed the -S-H site is chemically deactivated so that further conjugation with both bare Fe_3O_4 and Fe_3O_4-BSA Cs is prohibited. An important fact revealed by the data shown in Figs.5.21-5.22 is that the Fe_3O_4-BSA Cs are more effective candidates for the adsorption of Hcy by inhibiting the formation of the dimer homocystine, at least for the low Hcy concentration regime. In Fig.5.22(a) referring to $C_{Hcy} = 740$ μmol/L we see that the incubated Fe_3O_4-BSA Cs samples does not present discernible signatures for the formation of homocystine, whereas Fig.5.21(a) reveals that the incubated bare Fe_3O_4 sample of the same initial Hcy concentration clearly presents that homocystine are formed inhibiting their binding with bare Fe_3O_4 FNs.

From these NMR data a significant drawback of the TBS employed in the present book, namely BSA, is unveiled. In blood serum, TTSs that have high protein-binding affinity, such as Hcy, are already bound to proteins (mostly with HSA) so that their formerly active site has been chemically deactivated. Thus, regarding future *in vivo* applications, neither BSA nor HSA can serve as efficient TBS since they do not guaranty chemical reactivity higher than that of the protein that is already bound with the respective TTS. Antibodies are probably ideal TBS since either they can target different active sites of a TTS from the ones already occupied or they can substitute the protein that is already bound with the TTS owing to the relatively higher affinity of the antibodies. This issue is also discussed in Chapter (7).

These findings are not observed only in the ^{1}H NMR data but are further supported by

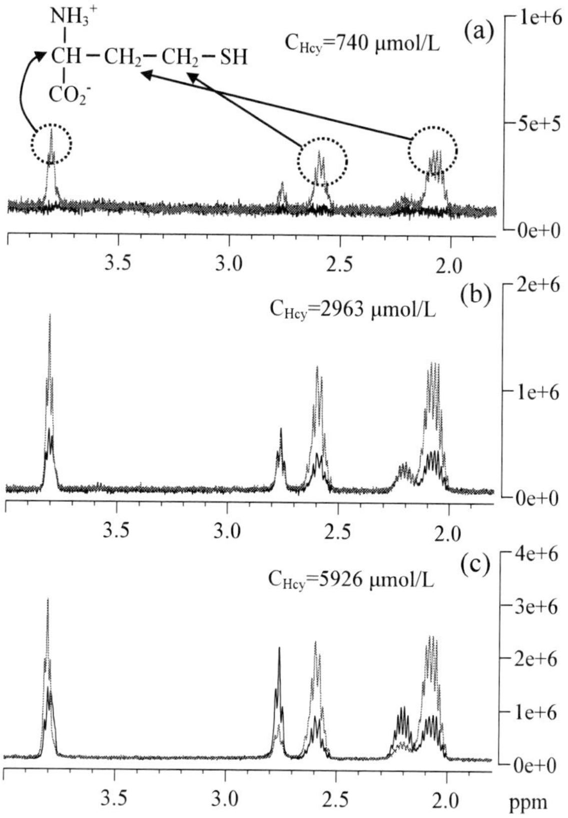

Figure 5.20. Comparative ^{1}H NMR spectra for the determination of the Hcy concentration remaining in the supernatant after its reaction with Fe_3O_4-BSA Cs. Black curves correspond to the supernatant drawn from each sample after Hcy has been adsorbed onto the FNs, while grey (red) curves correspond to the respective reference Hcy solutions having the same concentrations of (a) $C_{Hcy} = 740$, (b) 2963, and (c) 5926 μmol/L. In these experiments the FNs concentration was $C_{FNs} = 50$ mmol/L.

UV-VIS results. Representative UV-VIS data are shown in Figs.5.23(a)-5.23(c) for freshly prepared, incubated and naturally maturated (without incubation) samples, respectively. We see that both incubation and maturation promote the occurrence of an extra broad absorption peak that is centered at $245 - 250$ nm. By invoking standard knowledge on the formation of disulfide bonds and comparing with the ^{1}H NMR data we ascribe these newly evolving peaks to extra absorption coming from the formation of -S-S- disulfide bonds existing in homocystine.

Fluorescence Polarization Immunoassay method: Finally, the adsorption of Hcy onto Fe_3O_4 FNs and Fe_3O_4-BSA Cs was examined by the standard Fluorescence Polarization Immunoassay (FPIA) method that is routinely used in clinical practice for determining the concentration of tHcy. [135, 136] Briefly, the FPIA method relies on the reduction of the various oxidized Hcy forms, such as Hcy-S-S-Hcy, Hcy-S-S-Cys, and protein-Cy-S-S-Hcy complexes (see the discussion at the beginning of subsection "Evaluation of the toxin bind-

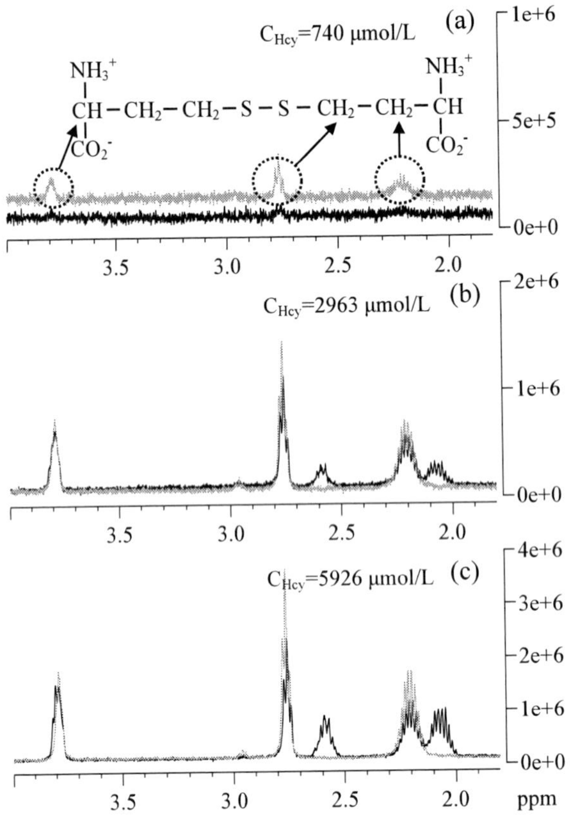

Figure 5.21. Comparative ^{1}H NMR spectra for the determination of the Hcy concentration remaining in the supernatant after its reaction with bare Fe_3O_4 FNs. Supernatant was drawn both when Fe_3O_4-Hcy samples were freshly prepared and when they were incubated for 12 hours. Black curves correspond to the freshly prepared samples, while grey (green) curves correspond to the incubated ones. Both series correspond to the same initial Hcy concentrations of (a) $C_{Hcy} = 740$, (b) 2963, and (c) 5926 μmol/L. In these experiments the FNs concentration was $C_{FNs} = 50$ mmol/L.

ing affinity and capacity of bare FNs and FN-BSA Cs") by treatment with dithiothreitol (DTT) that breaks the existing disulfide bonds -S-S- so that fHcy is finally recovered. Subsequently, fHcy is transformed to S-adenosyl-L-homocysteine (SAH) following a highly selective enzyme conversion by means of SAH hydrolase and excessive adenosine. Appropriate amounts of SAH and of a mouse monoclonal antibody are incubated for sufficient time, then a second SAH aliquot and a fluoresceinated analog of SAH are added. Finally, the intensity of fluorescence polarized light is measured by means of a FPIA system so that the Hcy concentration is determined. [135, 136]

Table 5.2 presents the results that were obtained for the same samples for which the UV-VIS and ^{1}H NMR data were presented above. The results refer to the initial values of Hcy concentration and the remaining ones in the supernatant after the bare Fe_3O_4 FNs and the Fe_3O_4-BSA Cs were retracted by means of a magnetic field. We see that the Hcy

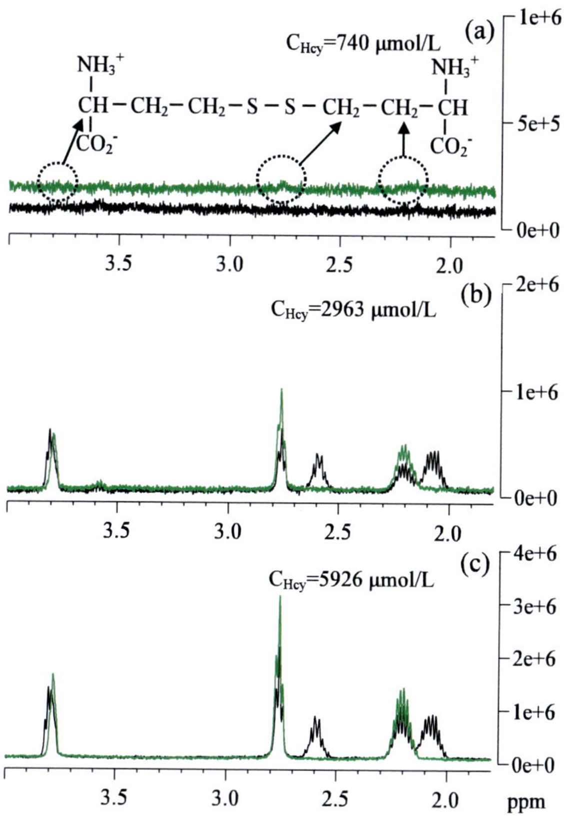

Figure 5.22. Comparative ^{1}H NMR spectra for the determination of the Hcy concentration remaining in the supernatant after its reaction with Fe_3O_4-BSA Cs. Supernatant was drawn both when Fe_3O_4-Hcy samples were freshly prepared and when they were incubated for 12 hours. Black curves correspond to the freshly prepared samples, while grey (green) curves correspond to the incubated ones. Both series correspond to the same initial Hcy concentrations of (a) $C_{Hcy} = 740$, (b) 2963, and (c) 5926 μmol/L. In these experiments the FNs concentration was $C_{FNs} = 50$ mmol/L.

concentration remaining in the supernatant is strongly reduced when compared to its initial value obviously owing to the adsorption of Hcy onto bare Fe_3O_4 FNs and Fe_3O_4-BSA Cs. These data are plotted in Fig.5.24(c) right below where the results obtained with the three different techniques are discussed comparatively.

Discussion of the results obtained on Hcy: Here we discuss some important issues on the overall applicability of the proposed MAHD method for the removal of Hcy. First, let us comparatively present the results obtained by the three different techniques employed in our work, namely UV-VIS, NMR and FPIA. In Figs.5.24(a)-5.24(c) we present the dependence of the Hcy concentration remaining in the supernatant on the initial Hcy value for bare Fe_3O_4 FNs (solid circles) and Fe_3O_4-BSA Cs (open circles). Panel (a) refers to the results obtained with UV-VIS spectrophotometry, panel (b) shows the results coming from ^{1}H NMR spectroscopy, and panel (c) the ones obtained with the FPIA method. *Despite*

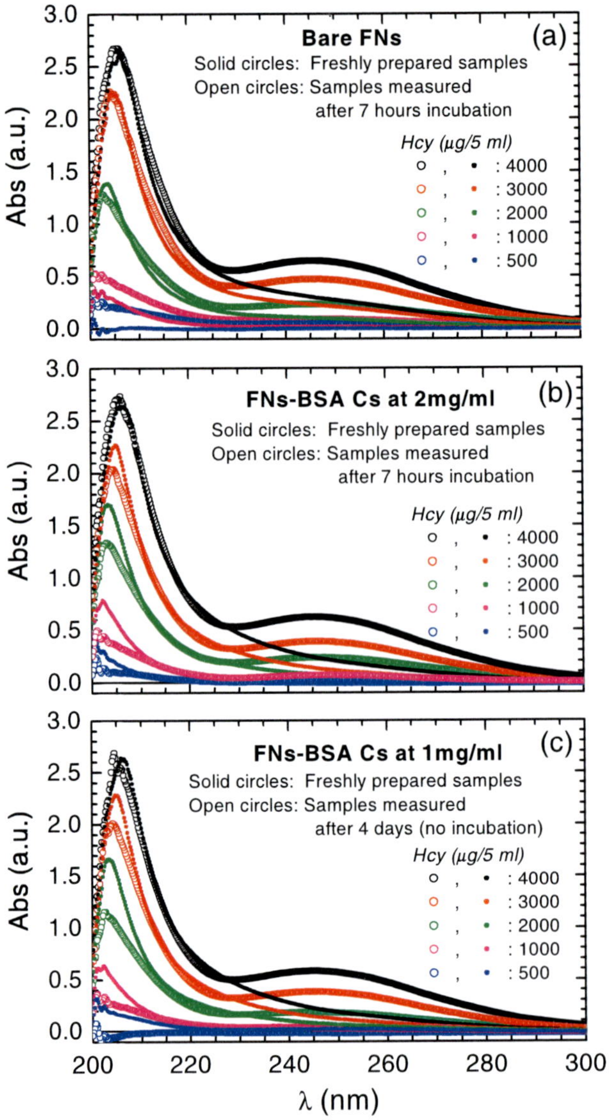

Figure 5.23. UV-VIS absorption data (focused in the range of 200 – 300 nm) revealing the maturation process of various FN-BSA Cs that were prepared at different BSA content of the host solution, when incubated: (a) 0 mg/mL (bare FNs) and (b) 2 mg/mL, and (c) without being incubated for 1 mg/mL. Different cases of systematically increasing amounts of Hcy are presented ranging from 500 to 4000 $\mu g/5$ mL. Small solid circles represent data obtained in the freshly prepared samples, while large open circles correspond to the maturated samples.

some quantitative differences, that should be expected, the experimental data obtained with all three techniques exhibit excellent qualitative agreement. We clearly see that there is a threshold value of the initial Hcy concentration, that slightly exceeds $C_{Hcy} = 740$ μmol/L, below which almost all Hcy is adsorbed onto both bare Fe_3O_4 FNs and Fe_3O_4-BSA Cs.

Table 5.2. Initial and remaining Hcy concentration upon adsorption onto bare Fe_3O_4 FNs and Fe_3O_4-BSA Cs

	Bare FNs	FN-BSA Cs
Initial (μmol/L)	*Remaining* (μmol/L)	*Remaining* (μmol/L)
0	0	0
148	2.2	1.7
296	3.4	2.4
740	16.9	18.3
1481	116.3	194.5
2963	558.0	534.6
4444	1028.2	977.1
5926	1480.8	1377.5

Above 740 μmol/L free Hcy is revealed in the supernatant a fact that indicates the saturation of the FN-BSA Cs binding capacity. Furthermore we see that for relatively high Hcy concentration the binding capacity of Fe_3O_4-BSA Cs is higher when compared to the capacity of bare Fe_3O_4 FNs. This observation relates to the fact that Hcy has high protein-binding affinity and confirms our former expectation that BSA could be an efficient TBS candidate.

The results presented up to now are quite impressive regarding the binding affinity and capacity of both bare Fe_3O_4 FNs and Fe_3O_4-BSA Cs for Hcy. However, these results should be subjected to more strict criticism. The concentration of FNs used in these experiments is relatively high (50 mmol/L). In future *in vivo* applications in animal models, significantly lower doses should be administered comparable to the ones that are routinely used in clinical practice so that the possibility of serious side effects to be minimized. Extended knowledge on these topics coming from the treatment of iron-deficiency anemia in both non-HD and HD dependent CKD patients could be enlightening for guiding our efforts. For instance, one of the iron agents that is most commonly used in clinical practice is Venofer® that is an aqueous iron(III) hydroxide-sucrose complex for intravenous administration. [58] One 5-mL vial of Venofer® provides 100 mg of iron that is the well established recommended dose administered to ESRD patients during a single HD session for the treatment of iron deficiency anemia. [137] Thus, the effective blood concentration of iron after administration of a 5-mL vial of Venofer® amounts to 15 mg/L when we assume that the blood content is approximately 8% of the total body weight of an 80 Kg patient. This concentration is far below the well accepted safety dose so that possible side effects are almost negligible. [58, 137]

In our *in vitro* experiments on the adsorption of Hcy we used Fe_3O_4 FNs at a concentration of 0.25 mmol/5 mL (58 mg/5 mL) which amounts to 50 mmol/L (11.6 g/L). This iron concentration is extremely high and completely unacceptable for being used in *in vivo* applications. *Nevertheless, in our in vitro experiments we have preliminarily used such high concentrations of Fe_3O_4 FNs in order to raise the impressive adsorption of comparably extreme amounts of Hcy onto them.*

Ultimately, in order to explore the possibility of future *in vivo* applications significantly

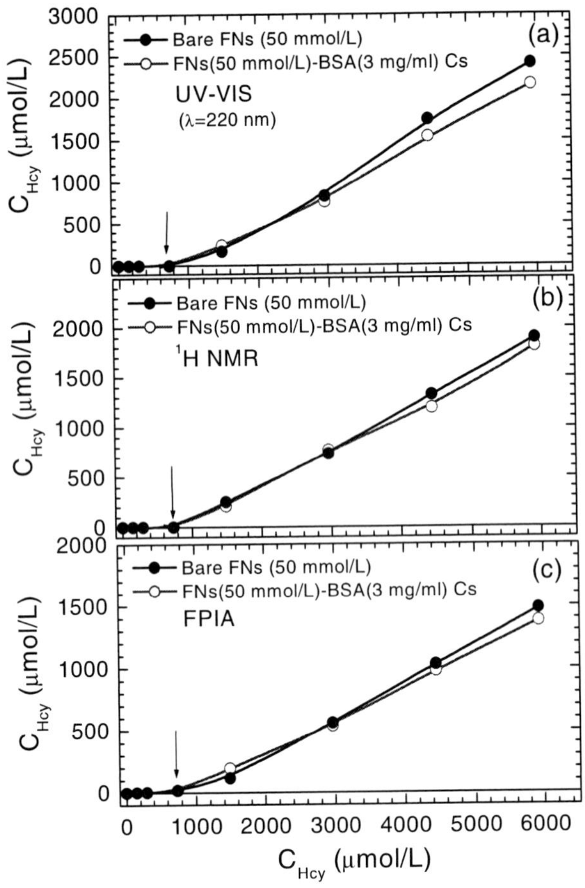

Figure 5.24. Comparison of the Hcy concentration remaining in the supernatant of bare FNs (solid circles) and FN-BSA Cs prepared under 3 mg/mL content of BSA (open circles) that were progressively loaded with Hcy, as they were determined by means of (a) UV-VIS absorption data obtained at $\lambda = 220$ nm, (b) ^{1}H NMR measurements, and (c) standard FPIA biochemical methods. In all these experiments the FNs concentration was $C_{FNs} = 50$ mmol/L.

lower concentrations of bare Fe_3O_4 FNs and Fe_3O_4-BSA Cs should be employed. To this end we performed systematic UV-VIS experiments by keeping constant the concentration of Hcy and varying the concentration of Fe_3O_4 FNs. Detailed UV-VIS results were obtained for sample series having the initial concentration of $C_{Hcy} = 200$, 130 and 50 μmol/L and progressively increasing concentration of bare Fe_3O_4 FNs ranging in $C_{FNs} = 0 - 50$ mmol/L. We have to note that the concentration of $C_{Hcy} = 200$ μmol/L is well inside the regime of severe hyperhomocysteinemia, while the one of $C_{Hcy} = 50$ μmol/L falls in the upper limit of intermediate hyperhomocysteinemia (see Table 5.1).

The evaluation of these UV-VIS data enabled us to determine the gradual reduction of the Hcy concentration upon its adsorption onto bare Fe_3O_4 FNs. The obtained data are shown in Fig.5.25 where we present the dependence of the Hcy concentration remaining in the supernatant on the progressively increasing Fe_3O_4 FNs concentration. These data reveal that relatively low concentrations of Fe_3O_4 FNs can easily handle cases of intermediate hyperhomocysteinemia since by using $C_{FNs} = 3$ mmol/L we are able to reduce Hcy from $C_{Hcy} = 50$ μmol/L to below 10 μmol/L (see the curve referring to $C_{Hcy} = 50$ μmol/L).

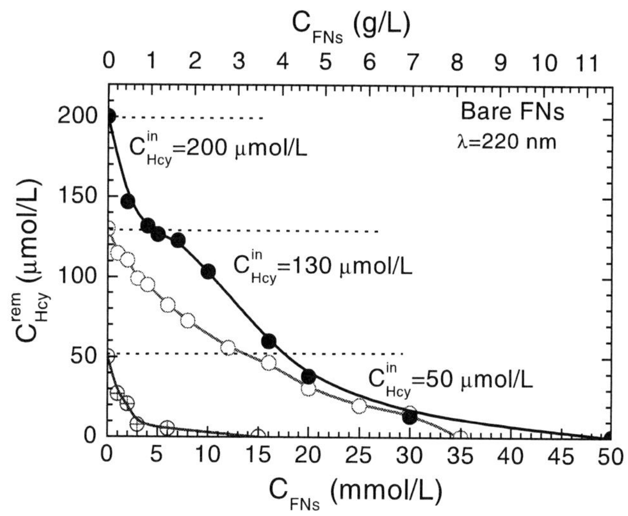

Figure 5.25. Concentration of Hcy remaining in the supernatant, C^{rem}_{Hcy} after its reaction with bare Fe_3O_4 FNs as it is determined from UV-VIS data taken at $\lambda = 220$ nm. Three sets of data are presented for different initial concentrations of Hcy ranging from intermediate to severe hyperhomocysteinemia. Each set has the same initial Hcy concentration, C^{in}_{Hcy} and refers to progressively increasing concentration of bare Fe_3O_4 FNs, C_{FNs}.

Currently, first-line strategies for the normalization of tHcy rely on supplementation of folate, B_{12}, and B_6 vitamins, betaine, serine, creatine. [113–116, 122, 123] Also, dialysis with high-flux filters has also been employed. [122] However, many cases of not only severe hyperhomocysteinemia but also of mild hyperhomocysteinemia (see Table 5.1) cannot be handled adequately so that a significant patients population does not respond to these strategies. [114–116, 122, 123] The *in vitro* results that are presented in Fig.5.25 reveal the possibility for an alternative way for the treatment of hyperhomocysteinemia in ESRD patients. Also, we have to note that the benefits of this new method could be very important and cannot be estimated at the moment without having at hand results coming from *in vivo* applications. In contrast to the practice of B vitamin agents administration where Hcy is either reformed to methionine under the action of B_{12}-dependent methionine synthase, or transformed to Cys following an alternative B_6-dependent biochemical pathway, our method *enables the complete removal of this toxin from the patient.*

2.2.2. p-Cresol

As a second model toxin for demonstrating the *in vitro* applicability of MAHD we have chosen a compound belonging to the group of cresols, namely p-Cresol (pC) that has the formula $(CH_3)C_6H_4(OH)$, MW$=$ 108.1 D and the respective structure that is schematically shown in Fig.5.26. pC is also termed as 4−methylphenol and *para*-cresol. Generally, cresols are aromatic organic compounds that result from phenols by substitution of a methyl group onto the benzene ring. Specifically, pC is constructed by a hydroxyl and a methyl groups that reside at two exact opposite sites on a benzene ring.

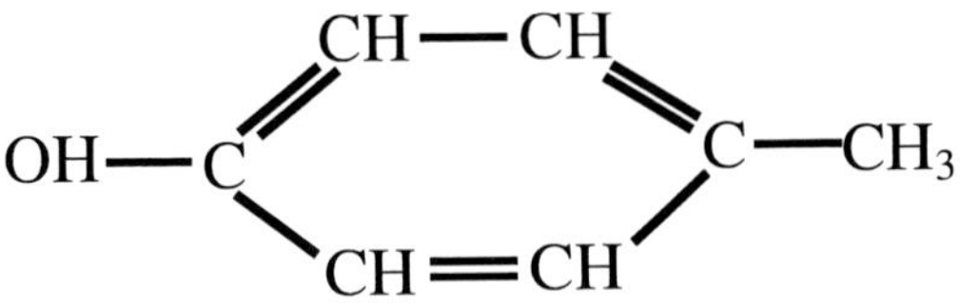

pC

Figure 5.26. Schematic illustration of the structure of pC.

Regarding its occurrence in human individuals, pC originates naturally in the intestine from the metabolism of two amino acids, namely tyrosine and phenylalanine. In CKD patients the pC serum concentration is elevated [138] inhibiting important metabolic processes that are related to free radicals production by activated phagocytes. [19, 84]

Generally, pC was selected as the second favorable TTS for demonstrating the *in vitro* applicability of MAHD for the following basic reasons: First, its significant biological impact on various metabolic processes. [19, 84] Second, the inability of conventional HD therapy to remove efficiently this toxin owing to its protein binding affinity. [19, 84] Third, apart from its protein binding affinity, the lipophilic nature of pC is incompatible with the purely hydrophilic dialysates that are routinely used in HD practice. Thus, pC accumulates in ESRD patients on HD. Table 5.3 summarizes normal and pathological pC concentrations that are met in ESRD patients. [20] As an overall consequence of the second and third reasons the removal of pC by conventional HD does not correlate with the removal of classical markers such as urea and creatinine [139] thus making the estimation of its removal adequacy more complex. Alternative strategies that have been currently introduced for the removal of phenols (the general category of compounds where pC can be classified) rely on HD against albumin-containing dialysates. [140, 141] Specifically, apart from the reasons mentioned above, Hcy was chosen as a favorable candidate TTS owing to the following technical ones: [34]

Table 5.3. Normal and pathological pC blood serum levels. [20]

Condition	pC (mg/L)
Normal	< 1
Intermediate	20
Severe	40

(i) The hydroxyl group residing at one site of the benzene ring should exhibit high chemical reactivity even with the bare Fe_3O_4 FNs.

(ii) As mentioned above it is well known that pC has high affinity to binding with proteins. Thus, in human individuals pC is mainly bound with HSA the most widely occurring protein in human serum. Furthermore, regarding the biological significance of pC, recently it has been shown that free pC (fpC) rather than total pC (tpC) mainly exerts toxicity in uremic individuals. [85] In Ref. [85] it was also shown that fpC depends on both tpC and HSA serum concentration, so that hypoalbuminemia is related with increased fpC fraction and higher toxicity. Given the close structural relation between HSA and BSA we expected that, similarly to HSA, BSA could efficiently bind with pC so that the Fe_3O_4-BSA Cs should exhibit higher binding capacity for this TTS when compared to the bare Fe_3O_4 FNs. Thus, the BSA part of the Cs could serve as an efficient TBS to conjugate and eventually remove fpC so that its toxic action to be minimized. Ultimately, since protein-bound pC probably has a secondary toxic influence (see Ref. [85] and references therein) an efficient way should be found so that also protein-bound pC to be conjugated and ultimately removed. To that end, more sophisticated TBSs should be employed, such as pC antibodies, for the efficient conjugation with already protein-bound pC (either by replacing the protein part of the already formed pC-protein conjugates or by binding with pC through other active sites).

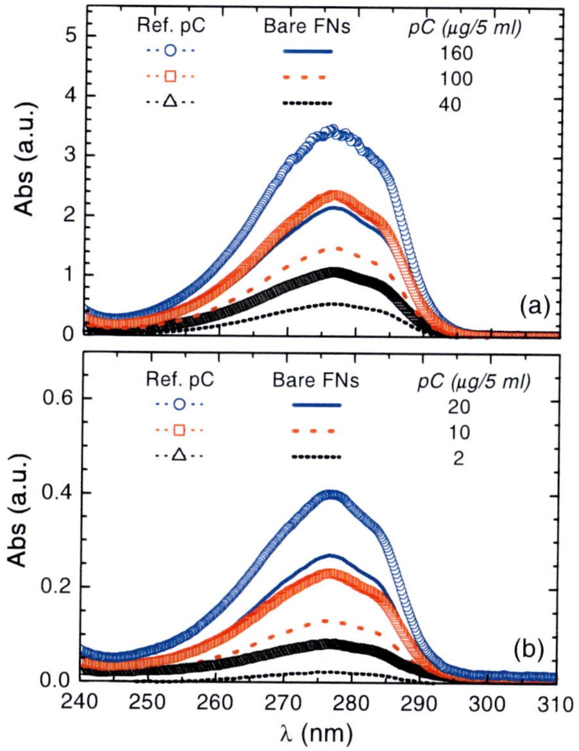

Figure 5.27. UV-VIS absorption data (focused in the range of 240 − 310 nm) for the supernatant that was drawn after the reaction of pC with bare Fe_3O_4 FNs for (a) high, and (b) low pC concentrations ranging in 2 to 160 $\mu g/5$ mL (line curves). For the sake of comparison, in all cases the data obtained in the respective reference pC solution are shown (open symbols).

UV-VIS spectrophotometry: Figures 5.27(a)-5.27(b) and 5.28(a)-5.28(b) present systematic UV-VIS absorption results obtained in the supernatant that was drawn from samples after the reaction of pC with bare Fe_3O_4 FNs and Fe_3O_4-BSA Cs, respectively. We recall that after their preparation the Fe_3O_4-BSA Cs were washed adequately with saline in order excessive NH_4OH to be removed. Finally, they were dispersed in saline so that the resulted suspension has pH= 6.5. Afterwards, pC was added and adequate stirring follows (for a couple of minutes) without any further treatment. Routinely, after waiting for an hour we retract the Fe_3O_4-BSA Cs by means of an externally applied magnetic field and the supernatant was drawn. The UV-VIS absorption data obtained for each supernatant provide information for the remaining concentration of pC by performing a direct comparison with the relative curve obtained on the respective reference pC solution. A practical issue of technical interest that should be clearly mentioned here is that in these UV-VIS measurements as baseline we used the supernatant of the respective pC-free bare Fe_3O_4 FNs or Fe_3O_4-BSA Cs sample that it was prepared following the same preparation conditions. Thus, all the curves measured in each series reveal exclusively the remaining concentration of pC in the supernatant.

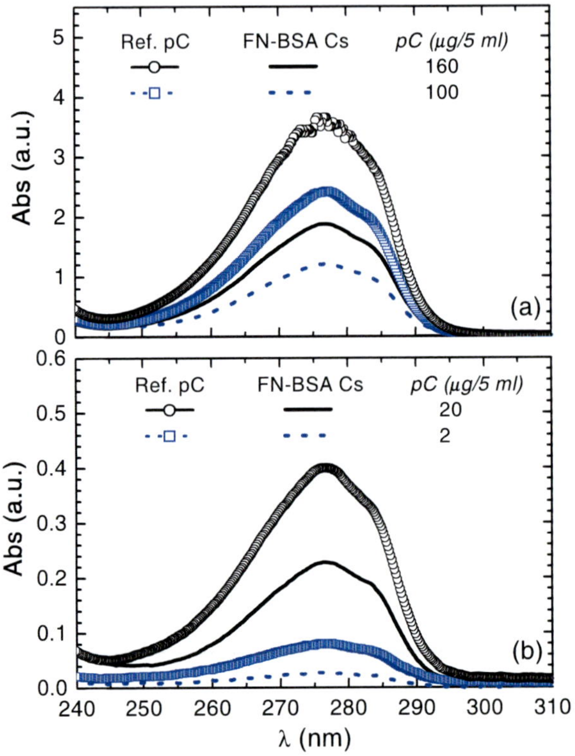

Figure 5.28. UV-VIS absorption data (focused in the range of 240 − 310 nm) for the supernatant that was drawn after the reaction of pC with Fe_3O_4-BSA Cs prepared at 3 mg/mL BSA content, for (a) high, and (b) low pC concentrations ranging in 2 to 160 μg/5 mL (line curves). For the sake of comparison, in all cases the data obtained in the respective reference pC solution are shown (open symbols).

In Figs.5.27(a)-5.27(b) and 5.28(a)-5.28(b) we show the curves obtained in the supernatant of samples after the reaction of pC with bare Fe_3O_4 or Fe_3O_4-BSA Cs, and all respective reference curves for pC concentration ranging up to 160 μg/5 mL (32 mg/L). Thus, the pC concentration range studied here is well inside the pathological values that are routinely observed in ESRD patients on HD therapy (see Table 5.3). [20] From the data presented in Figs.5.27(a)-5.27(b) and 5.28(a)-5.28(b) we can see that after pC has reacted with both bare Fe_3O_4 FNs and Fe_3O_4-BSA Cs the remaining concentration in the supernatant reduces strongly when compared with the initial value. *Proving our former expectation, these systematic data reveal that pC reacts intensively with both bare Fe_3O_4 FNs (Figs.5.27(a)-5.27(b)) and Fe_3O_4-BSA Cs (Figs.5.28(a)-5.28(b)).*

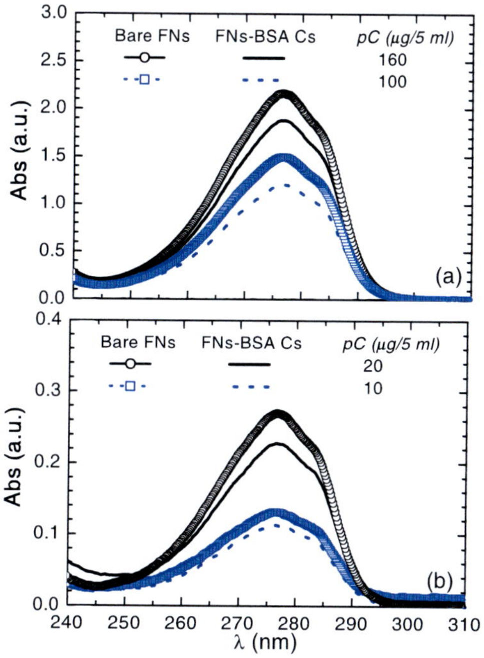

Figure 5.29. Comparative UV-VIS absorption data (focused in the range of 240 – 310 nm) for the supernatant that was drawn after the reaction of pC with bare Fe_3O_4 (open points) and Fe_3O_4-BSA Cs prepared at 3 mg/mL BSA content (line curves), for (a) high and (b) low pC concentrations ranging in 10 to 160 μg/5 mL.

Furthermore, the presence of BSA as TBS clearly increase the binding capacity of Fe_3O_4-BSA Cs when compared to bare Fe_3O_4 FNs. Comparative UV-VIS data for the two cases are presented in Figs.5.29(a)-5.29(b). We clearly see that in all cases the absorption curves obtained for Fe_3O_4-BSA Cs are placed slightly below or even well below the respective ones obtained for bare Fe_3O_4 FNs. *This experimental fact proves our former expectation that the Fe_3O_4-BSA Cs should have higher binding capacity owing to the protein-binding affinity of pC.* A note of some interest is that the binding dynamics of Fe_3O_4-BSA Cs with pC, in contrast to what was observed for the case of Hcy, is rather slow. This is a strong disadvantage of the specific TBS, namely BSA used in the present project. This disadvantage should be resolved in future studies by using more sophisticated TBSs.

Table 5.4. Normal and pathological β2-m blood serum levels. [20]

Condition	β2-m (mg/L)
Normal	< 2
Intermediate	50
Severe	100

2.2.3. β2-microglobulin

As a third model toxin we have chosen β2-microglobulin (β2-m). [36] This toxin is significantly more complex [142–144] when compared to both Hcy and pC. β2-m, a middle-MW compound, MW= 11818 D, is currently identified as a relatively important toxin that interferes with many biological processes. High concentrations of β2-m in blood serum is associated with formation of amyloid fibrils that deposit on ligaments, tendons and joints resulting in disorders of bones. [28, 29, 90, 145–147] Also, these fibrils are deposited to the digestive system and heart, leading to premature atherosclerosis and CVD. [28,29,90, 145–147] Generally speaking, the disorder motivated by the deposition of amyloid fibrils is called amyloidosis. Regarding ESRD patients on HD, nowadays it well known that low-flux dialysers are not able to efficiently replace the filtering and excretion ability of kidney for β2-m. High-flux dialysers have been employed for the more efficient removal of β2-m. However, many recent studies have revealed that HD based on high-flux dialysers is also not adequate for the normalization of β2-m blood serum levels. [147–152] Thus, when referring to ESRD patients on HD, the disorder motivated by the deposition of amyloid fibrils is called dialysis-related amyloidosis [28, 29, 90, 145–152] owing to the inefficiency of conventional HD to remove β2-m. Table 5.4 summarizes normal and pathological β2-m blood serum concentrations that are met in ESRD patients. [20]

The importance of RRF on the removal of many middle-MW toxins has been evidenced. Referring to β2-m, Farrington and colleagues have recently shown that the contribution of even extremely low RRF of 1 mL/min is beneficial for its removal. [151] Thus, modern trends suggest that preservation of RRF should be an objective so that the efficient removal of middle-MW toxins, such as β2-m, to be assisted. A novel strategy that also has been employed, at an experimental stage, for preventing the onset or progression of dialysis-related amyloidosis relies on intracorporeal cell implantation by using proximal tubular endocytic receptors that mediate both cellular uptake and degradation of β2-m. [152]

From the discussion made above it becomes clear that dialysis-related amyloidosis [28, 29, 90, 145–147] is a disorder that currently cannot be treated adequately, motivating serious health complications mainly related to CVD. Thus, β2-m was selected for demonstrating the *in vitro* applicability of MAHD for the reasons discussed above: First, its significant biological impact for ESRD patients. Second, the inability of conventional low- and high-flux dialysers to efficiently remove this toxin, owing to its protein-binding affinity. For the quantitative determination of β2-m we employed UV-VIS spectrophotometry, CD spectropolarimetry and an Turbidimetry Immunoassay method that is most commonly used in clinical practice.

UV-VIS spectrophotometry: We first discuss the UV-VIS absorption data. During these experiments the Fe_3O_4 FNs and the Fe_3O_4-BSA Cs were redispersed in saline so that pH= 6.5 was achieved. Subsequently, β2-m was added at a desired concentration (the studied concentrations range from normal levels to severe conditions, see Table 5.4) and adequate stirring followed for a couple of minutes without any further treatment. Routinely, after 30 min the supernatant was drawn under magnetic retraction of the Cs so as the remaining concentration of β2-m was determined by means of UV-VIS spectrophotometry. A practical issue of technical interest that should be clearly mentioned here is that in these UV-VIS measurements as baseline we used the supernatant of the respective β2-m-free bare Fe_3O_4 FNs or Fe_3O_4-BSA Cs sample that it was prepared following the same preparation conditions. Thus, all the curves measured in each series reveal exclusively the remaining concentration of β2-m in the supernatant.

Figures 5.30(a)-5.30(b) show representative UV-VIS data obtained for the supernatant that was drawn after the reaction of β2-m with bare Fe_3O_4 FNs and Fe_3O_4-BSA Cs that were prepared at a BSA concentration of 2 and 4 mg/mL. These data refer to initial concentration of β2-m, $C^{in}_{\beta 2-m} = 20$ mg/L. The result coming from a reference β2-m solution of the same concentration 20 mg/L is also presented. In Fig. 5.30(a) we clearly see that when β2-m has reacted with bare Fe_3O_4 FNs and Fe_3O_4-BSA Cs, and subsequently these were magnetically retracted, there is no β2-m remaining in the supernatant, a proof that it has been completely adsorbed onto them. The results coming from CD spectropolarimetry (not shown) are consisted with the UV-VIS absorption ones. Figure 5.30(b) presents important data on the binding dynamics between bare Fe_3O_4 FNs and β2-m. These experiments were performed as follows: First, the supernatant of a bare Fe_3O_4 FNs sample was used for defining the baseline. Second, β2-m was added in the supernatant and the UV-VIS absorption was measured (thick black curve in Fig. 5.30(b)). Third, the FNs were redispersed in the vial under mild incubation for a desired duration. Fourth, the FNs were magnetically retracted and the supernatant was measured once again so that the remaining concentration of β2-m to be estimated. These data reveal that the reaction between β2-m and Fe_3O_4 FNs exhibits first-order dynamics since it proceeds rapidly, in a time scale of a few minutes. Accordingly, the results obtained on β2-m are even more impressive than the ones obtained for the binding dynamics between bare Fe_3O_4 FNs and Hcy where we observed that after $10-15$ min the reduction of the Hcy concentration was only $30-40\%$.

In the *in vitro* experiments presented in Figs. 5.30(a)-5.30(b) we used Fe_3O_4 FNs at an extremely high concentration of 58 mg/5 mL (11.6 g/L). This iron concentration cannot be used in future *in vivo* applications. In animal models, significantly lower doses should be administered, comparable to the ones that are routinely used for the treatment of iron-deficiency anemia. [58,137] Consequently, in order to explore the possibility of future *in vivo* applications, remarkably lower concentrations were used for bare Fe_3O_4 FNs and Fe_3O_4-BSA Cs, as we did for the case of Hcy. We prepared systematic series of samples by keeping constant the initial concentration of β2-m, $C^{in}_{\beta 2-m}$ and varying the concentration of Fe_3O_4 FNs, C_{FNs}. We have carefully surveyed both FNs and β2-m concentrations that range in the more realistic limits down to 46.4 mg/L (0.2 mmol/L) and 5 mg/L (0.423 μmol/L), respectively.

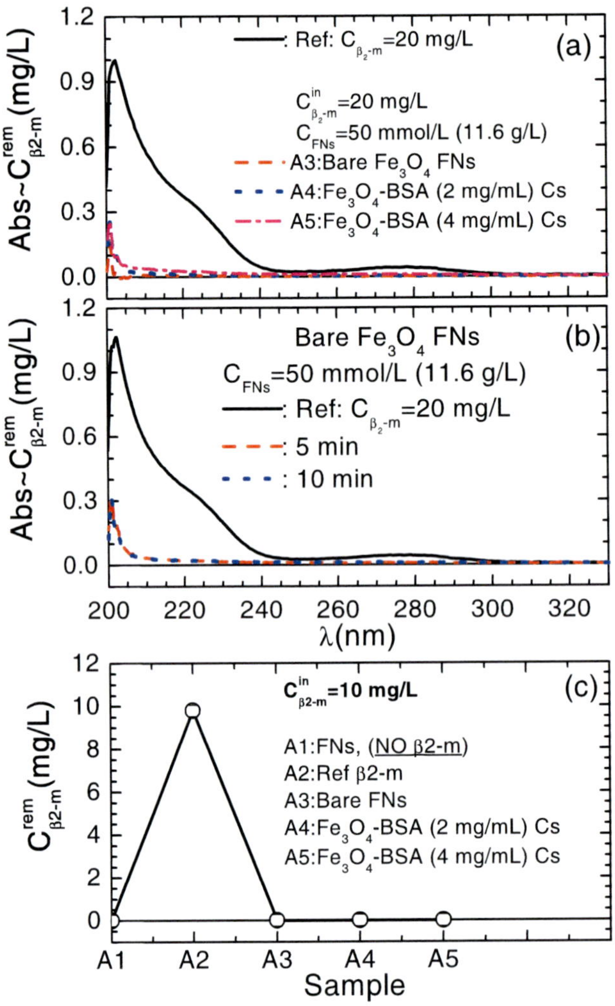

Figure 5.30. (a) UV-VIS absorption data obtained for the supernatant that was drawn after the reaction of β2-m with bare Fe_3O_4 FNs and Fe_3O_4-BSA Cs. These data reveal the reduction of the initial β2-m concentration, $C^{in}_{\beta2-m} = 20$ mg/L owing to its adsorption onto Fe_3O_4 FNs and Fe_3O_4-BSA Cs. The respective data for a reference β2-m solution having concentration 20 μg/mL are also shown. (b) UV-VIS data revealing the binding dynamics between β2-m and both Fe_3O_4 FNs and Fe_3O_4-BSA Cs (see text for details). (c) Concentration of β2-m remaining in the supernatant, $C^{rem}_{\beta2-m}$ as determined by the TIA method that is used in clinical practice. During these TIA experiments a β2-m-free supernatant drawn from bare Fe_3O_4 FNs (sample A1) has been tested to check that it consistently gives $C^{rem}_{\beta2-m} = 0$. In all these experiments the concentration of FNs was $C_{FNs} = 11.6$ g/L.

Figures 5.31(a)-5.31(b) present detailed UV-VIS absorption data showing the reduction of β2-m upon adsorption onto bare Fe_3O_4 FNs as their concentration, C_{FNs} progressively increases. Two series of samples are presented having initial β2-m concentration, $C^{in}_{\beta2-m} =$ 10 mg/L and 5 mg/L, respectively. The concentration of FNs in the two series ranges

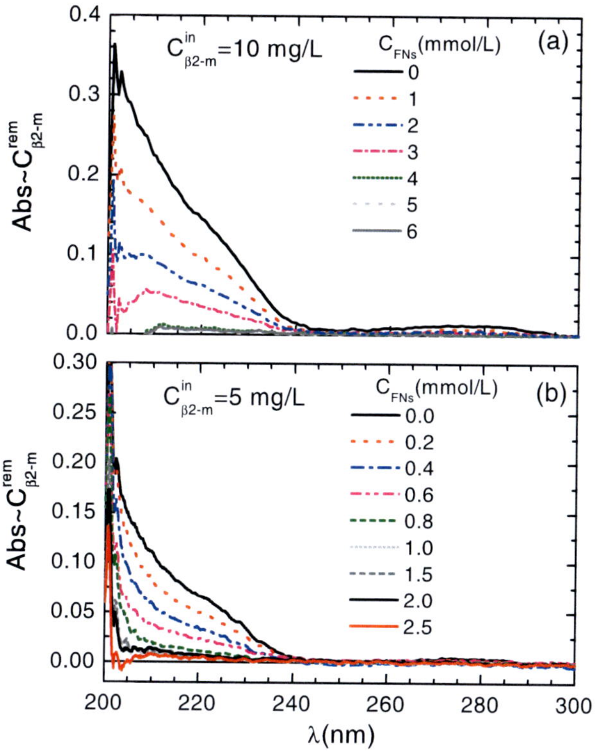

Figure 5.31. Detailed UV-VIS absorption data obtained in a sample series showing the reduction of the initial concentration of β2-m, $C^{in}_{\beta 2-m}$ upon adsorption onto bare Fe_3O_4 FNs as their concentration, C_{FNs} progressively increases. Two series of samples are shown having the same initial concentration (a) $C^{in}_{\beta 2-m} = 10$ mg/L, and (b) 5 mg/L.

in $0-6$ mmol/L and $0-2.5$ mmol/L, respectively. We see that as the concentration of FNs progressively increases the concentration of β2-m remaining in the supernatant $C^{rem}_{\beta 2-m}$ decreases in a monotonic way. These results clearly prove the ability of FNs to adsorb significant amounts of β2-m. The adsorption capacity is discussed below.

Turbidimetry Immunoassay method: For the verification of the UV-VIS and CD experimental results we have also employed a Turbidimetry Immunoassay (TIA) method that is commonly used in clinical practice for the determination of β2-m blood serum levels. Briefly, the quantitative determination of β2-m based on the TIA method was performed by using Quantia β2-m reagents on an Abbott AEROSET® platform. The Quantia β2-m reagents is a suspension of polystyrene latex particles of uniform size that are coated with the IgG fraction of an β2-m specific antibody. When a sample that contains β2-m is mixed with the reagent, complete conjugation between the β2-m specific antibody and β2-m takes place owing to their high affinity. The β2-m concentration is determined by means of a turbidimetry method. [153]

Figure 5.30(c) presents the results obtained with the TIA method for the same samples studied in Fig. 5.30(a) with UV-VIS absorption. The TIA results are consistent to the UV-VIS ones. Finally, we have to note that in these TIA experiments the supernatant drawn

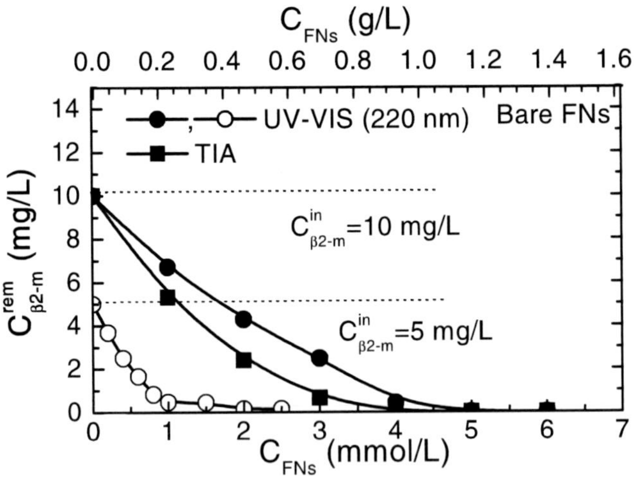

Figure 5.32. Concentration of the β2-m remaining in the supernatant, $C^{rem}_{\beta 2-m}$ after the reaction with bare Fe_3O_4 FNs as determined from the UV-VIS data shown in Figs. 5.31(a)-5.31(b) (at $\lambda = 220$ nm). The data refer to constant initial β2-m concentration, $C^{in}_{\beta 2-m}$ of 10 mg/L (solid circles) and 5 mg/L (open circles) and progressively increasing concentration of FNs, C_{FNs}. For the samples referring to 10 mg/L, $C^{rem}_{\beta 2-m}$ has also been determined by the TIA method (squares).

from a β2-m-free bare FNs sample (sample A1) has also been tested in order to confirm the reliability of the obtained results. This is absolutely needed in order to ensure that a negligible amount of FNs that could exist in the supernatant (after their magnetic retraction) does not interfere with the clinical method, giving erroneous results on the determination of $C^{rem}_{\beta 2-m}$.

Figure 5.32 summarizes the results presented in Figs. 5.31(a)-5.31(c). It shows the dependence of the β2-m concentration that remains in the supernatant, $C^{rem}_{\beta 2-m}$ upon variation of the Fe_3O_4 FNs concentration, C_{FNs}. Two sets of data are shown that refer to the same initial concentration of β2-m, $C^{in}_{\beta 2-m}$ of 10 mg/L (solid circles) and 5 mg/L (open circles). For the samples referring to 10 mg/L, $C^{rem}_{\beta 2-m}$ has also been determined by means of TIA (squares). We see that a FNs concentration of 1 mmol/L (232 mg/L) is adequate to eliminate an initial concentration of β2-m of 5 mg/L. Thus, these *in vitro* results suggest that the MAHD method is promising for the treatment of dialysis-related amyloidosis.

Chapter 6

Experimental Results Obtained on the Dialysis Machine

To evaluate the proposed MAHD method in comparison to conventional HD we performed mock-dialysis experiments on Hcy dissolved in saline. [37] In these mock-dialysis experiments we employed standard Hemophan low-flux membranes since such membranes exhibit insufficient removal of low- and middle-MW toxins that have high affinity for blood-serum proteins. The employed dialysate was standard bicarbonate that is routinely used in HD (Na 138 mmol/L, HCO_3 35 mmol/L, K 1.5 mmol/L, Ca 1.25 mmol/L, Mg 0.75 mmol/L). The dialysate flow rate was kept at 500 mL/min, while the saline flow rate (blood compartment) ranged in 100 – 250 mL/min.

1. Magnetic Retraction of Bare Fe_3O_4 FNs and Fe_3O_4-BSA Cs

We have carefully evaluated the magnetic retraction efficiency of both bare Fe_3O_4 FNs and Fe_3O_4-BSA Cs under flow rate conditions that are routinely used in HD practice. Accordingly, the magnetic retraction efficiency in these mock-dialysis experiments was evaluated as follows: In saline we added either bare Fe_3O_4 FNs or Fe_3O_4-BSA Cs (prepared at a relatively low BSA concentration of 2 mg/mL so that to be highly magnetic) at a concentration of 100 mg/L and we performed sequential circulations under a flow rate of 100 – 250 mL/min.

As a "magnetic dialyser" we employed an array of 10 – 15 permanent magnets placed along the extracorporeal circulation line of the dialysis machine as shown in Fig. 6.1(a). Figures 6.1(b)-6.1(c) focus on part of the employed array of magnets prior to the first circulation and after two complete circulations, respectively. In Fig. 6.1(c) we clearly see that intense magnetic field gradients that are mainly produced at the edges of the disc-shaped magnets (the maximum magnetic field value is in the range of 1000 – 2000 Oe) effectively retract these highly magnetic Cs. In agreement to our *in vitro* experiments performed in the laboratory, [34, 35] these mock-dialysis experiments [37] revealed that a high flow rate of 200 – 250 mL/min act against complete removal of the Fe_3O_4-BSA Cs. In contrast, a lower

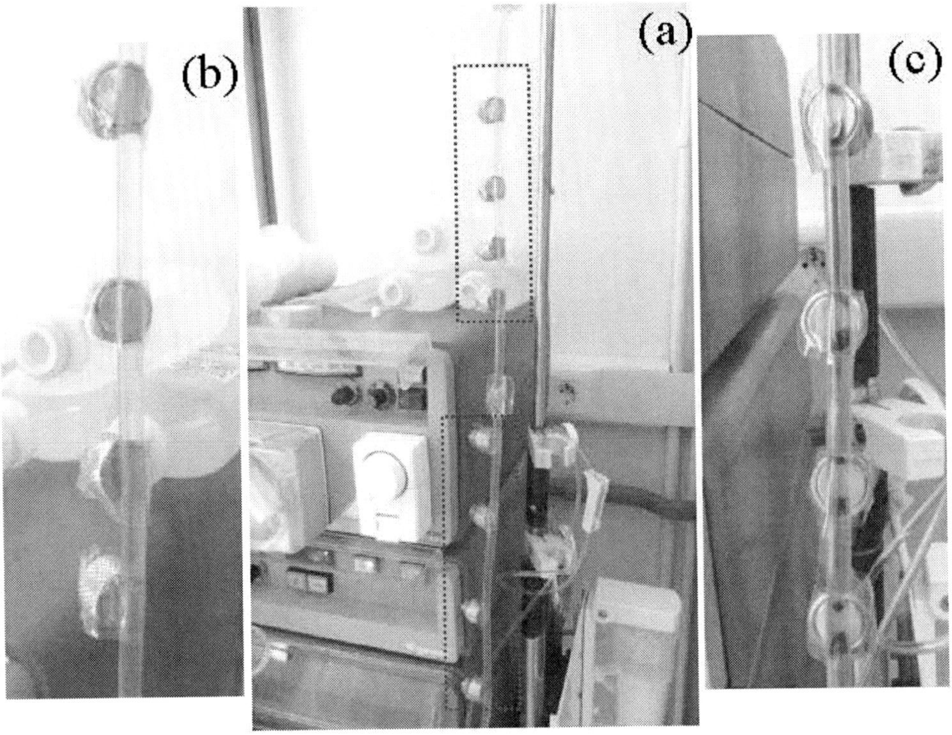

Figure 6.1. (a) Dialysis machine with a simple "magnetic dialyser" consisting of an array of permanent magnets placed along the extracorporeal circulation line. Detail of the array (b) prior to first circulation and (c) after two circulations, revealing the trapped Cs (dotted areas in (a)).

flow rate of 100 – 150 mL/min enables their almost complete retraction.

We note that after the end of the experiments we visually inspected the capillaries of the dialyser by means of a conventional stereoscope. Figures 6.2(a)-6.2(b) show representative images of the capillaries of a dialyser that was used in mock-dialysis experiments. Figure 6.2(a) shows the top view where the entry points of the capillaries are visible, while Fig. 6.2(b) presents the side view of capillaries that are placed close to the outer surface of the dialyser. We observed no evidence of agglomerated bare Fe_3O_4 or Fe_3O_4-BSA Cs at the surfaces of the capillaries. This clearly proves that the employed FNs do not chemically interact with the material of the capillaries. In agreement to this observation, we also had no indication of agglomerated bare Fe_3O_4 or Fe_3O_4-BSA Cs dispersed in the dialysate. *Thus, we may safely conclude that the employed bare* Fe_3O_4 *or* Fe_3O_4*-BSA Cs were removed from the extracorporeal blood circulation compartment under the action of the "magnetic dialyser" and not owing to diffusion/convection processes occurring at the capillaries of the conventional dialyser.*

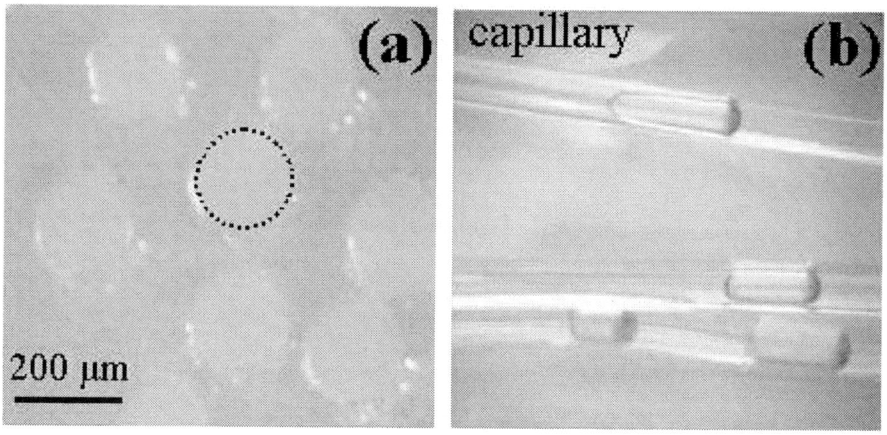

Figure 6.2. Representative images of the capillaries of a dialyser that was employed in MAHD mock-dialysis experiments for the evaluation of the magnetic retraction efficiency of Fe_3O_4-BSA Cs. (a) Top view of the capillaries' entry points. The bar represents 0.2 mm. (b) Side view of capillaries, along the flow direction.

2. Removal Efficiency of MAHD against Conventional HD for Hcy

The evaluation of the mock-dialysis applicability of MAHD was tested on Hcy. The MAHD mock-dialysis experiments were contrasted to conventional HD mock-dialysis ones. [37] During these MAHD mock-dialysis experiments Fe_3O_4 FNs or Fe_3O_4-BSA Cs were dispersed in 1 L saline at a typical concentration $C_{FNs} = 0.05$ mmol/L (11.6 mg/L). Hcy was added at a desired concentration ranging in 50 – 150 μmol/L and mild stirring followed for a couple of minutes without any further treatment. *We performed sequential mock-dialysis rounds with sampling at the end of each round.* The same procedure was followed in our reference conventional HD mock-dialysis experiments that were based on the standard low-flux dialyser without employing FNs and the "magnetic dialyser". In both experiments, the concentration of Hcy remaining in the supernatant was estimated by the standard FPIA method.

Figures 6.3(a)-6.3(b) show comparative data from these experiments. In the upper panel we present data for conventional HD experiments of initial Hcy concentration $C^{in}_{Hcy} = 62$ μmol/L (open circles) and MAHD experiments for initial Hcy concentration $C^{in}_{Hcy} = 100$ μmol/L and $C_{FNs} = 0.05$ mmol/L (solid circles). In both cases the data are normalized to the respective initial concentration of Hcy. We stress that in both MAHD and conventional HD experiments presented in Figs. 6.3(a)-6.3(b) the same flow rate of nominal value 220 mL/min was used in the saline compartment (blood compartment). The inset presents the respective percentage difference of the Hcy concentration between the conventional HD and the MAHD experiments. The lower panel shows in semilogarithmic plot, the variation of the Hcy concentration when normalized to the initial value of each experiment. In this plot, even the small differences existing at the end of the third and the fifth rounds of the MAHD and HD experiments become visible.

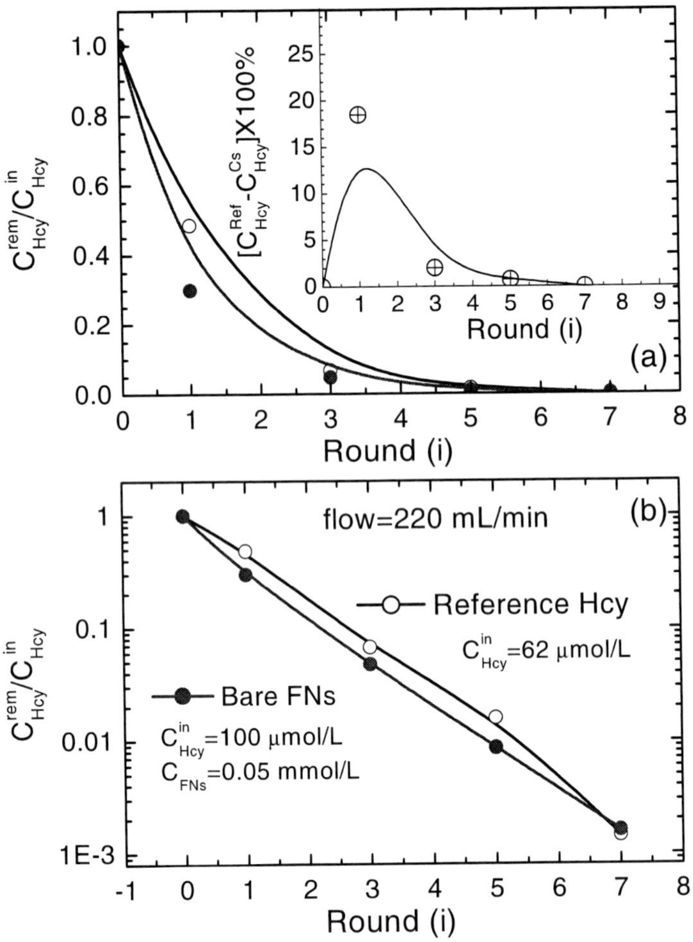

Figure 6.3. (a) Remaining concentration of Hcy (normalized to its initial value) after subsequent dialysis rounds. The reference HD experiments had initial Hcy concentration $C^{in}_{Hcy} = 62$ μmol/L (open circles), while the MAHD experiments on bare Fe_3O_4 FNs had initial Hcy concentration $C^{in}_{Hcy} = 100$ μmol/L and $C_{FNs} = 0.05$ mmol/L (solid circles). Both mock-dialysis experiments were performed at flow rate 220 mL/min. Inset presents the respective percentage difference of the Hcy concentration between conventional HD and MAHD experiments. (b) Semilogarithmic plot of the Hcy variation when normalized to the initial value of each experiment.

The presented data show clearly that, at early stages, MAHD shows a significantly higher decrease of the Hcy concentration when compared to reference HD. Despite the fact that after 7 circulations both MAHD and HD have successfully removed all Hcy content, the MAHD method obviously records a significantly higher overall removal efficiency since in this experiment the initial Hcy concentration was 66% higher when compared to the one of the reference HD ($C^{in}_{Hcy} = 100$ μmol/L and 62 μmol/L for MAHD and conventional HD experiments, respectively). We also stress that the nominal Fe_3O_4 concentration used in these mock-dialysis experiments typically amounts to 0.05 mmol/L (11.6 mg/L). This value is inside the well-established safety levels referring to the treatment of iron-deficiency anemia. [58, 137] Thus, the nominal Fe_3O_4 concentrations used in our mock-dialysis experiments will possibly enable future *in vivo* applications for the evaluation of MAHD in animal models.

Chapter 7

Conclusions and Perspectives

Late epidemiological studies reveal that the coexistence of HT, DM and HC are routinely met in a great percentage of elder individuals. Some studies estimate the prevalence in the USA as being up to 25% of the general population. These disorders, namely HT, DM and HC affect intensively the vascular network of the kidney so that early or established CKD is a disorder that inflicts many dietary restrictions in elder people that as a consequence further degrade the overall health status of the patient. Early detection and successful control of these disorders will possibly enable CKD patients to avoid ESRD. Unfortunately, ESRD relates to an important percentage of patients who have all the disorders associated with the MS. Other diseases that progressively damage kidney, thus leading to CKD, are Polycystic Kidney Disease (whether dominant or recessive), glomerulonephritis, chronic pyelonephritis etc. However, the synergy of HT, DM and HC is responsible for almost 75% of all adult cases. The community of patients that are subjected to permanent HD has been greatly expanded; it seems that owing to its connection with the MS nowadays ESRD gradually takes almost epidemic characteristics. Unfortunately, owing to the expanded patients population in many cases constraints on the resources inhibit the adequate dose of HD therapy that should be delivered to each individual. Inadequate HD dose is surely related to higher morbidity and mortality.

This is why we believe that our proposal [34–37] could be very important; hopefully, owing to the decrease of each dialysis session duration and the increased dialysis dose delivered to the patient our scientific outcome could possibly turn conventional HD that currently mainly serves as an expensive life-saving renal replacement therapy, to MAHD, a low-cost therapy that could significantly improve both the patient's quality-of-life and survival.

1. Extracorporeal MAHD

The newly introduced MAHD concept could trigger the scientific community to explore other more sophisticated and less invasive strategies that could also be based on utilization of FNs in HD. For instance, such a non-invasive strategy could rely on the entirely extracorporeal usage of FN-TBS Cs. According to this scenario the FN-TBS Cs should be injected at an entry point of the extracorporeal blood circulation line, thus having the opportunity to conjugate with the desired TTS only within a short period of time, during which blood flows along the circulation line. Accordingly, the FN-TBS-TTS Cs would be retracted at an exit point of the extracorporeal blood circulation line by means of a "magnetic dialyser" without being injected into the patient. This scenario, which could be termed Extracorporeal MAHD (EMAHD), is very attractive since the extracorporeal usage of FNs ensures negligible side effects.

However, from a technical point of view the realization of the EMAHD concept seems more complex when compared to MAHD once all other parameters that are routinely involved in HD therapy are considered. For instance, depending on the hemodynamic status of the patient the employed blood flow rates range in 200 – 350 mL/min. These values are relatively high. Also, the length of the blood circulation line should be minimum once this, among with the volume of the dialyser's blood compartment, define the total blood volume that circulates extracorporeally; obviously in order hemodynamic instabilities and hypotensive events to be avoided the extracorporeal total blood volume should be minimum. Commercially available blood circulation lines and dialysers that are routinely used in HD practice have such dimensions that the extracorporeal total blood volume does not exceed 200 mL. Once these parameters are taken into account we can estimate the period of time available for the accomplishment of the conjugation between the FN-TBS Cs and the TTS. This duration is strictly limited by the time needed for the Cs to flow along the extracorporeal blood circulation line since according to the EMAHD concept their utilization is entirely extracorporeal. By simple calculations we conclude that the available time duration for the conjugation to be accomplished is 1 min in the case where a blood flow rate of 200 mL/min is used. This is an extremely low conjugation time period that could be achieved only by uncommonly rapid chemical reactions that exhibit extreme first order binding dynamics.

However, one could invoke that, alternatively, an appropriately modified blood circulation line could be constructed so that the extracorporeal blood flow duration is increased, thus matching the realistic values needed for the respective binding reaction between the FN-TBS Cs and the TTS. By assuming that a time period of 5 min is needed for realistic binding to be accomplished, we conclude that the extracorporeal total blood volume is of the order of 1000 mL (in the case where a blood flow rate of 200 mL/min is employed). According to basic HD practice this value is unacceptably high.

Thus, we conclude that the possibility of the EMAHD method, at least as approached right above, is restricted by serious safety complications that conflict with standard HD practice.

2. MAHD

Returning to the MAHD method, in this book we have employed Fe_3O_4 FNs owing to their biocompatibility as the host carriers and a simple protein, BSA as the TBS part for the preparation of Cs. BSA is employed to further improve the biocompatibility of the FNs and most importantly to increase both the binding affinity and capacity for specific toxins that have protein-binding affinity. A detailed structural/morphological and magnetic evaluation of these Cs was presented. We presented *in vitro* experiments for the evaluation of the magnetic retraction efficiency and binding affinity and capacity of both bare Fe_3O_4 FNs and Fe_3O_4-BSA Cs for specific TTSs, namely Hcy, pC and β2-m. The obtained results prove that such FN-TBS Cs can be used for the purposes described in this book, since these well-known toxins of high biological significance, are drastically adsorbed on both bare FNs and FN-BSA Cs. The revealing result is that Hcy and β2-m are adsorbed not only in significant amounts but also very rapidly onto the carriers. Such a rapid binding reaction clearly proves that FNs could be employed in *in vivo* applications since the whole MAHD concept is based on the administration of the FN-TBS Cs timely prior to the HD session. Thus, the Cs are able to achieve the desired goal, that is to bind with the desired TTSs, during a small time period without triggering the immune system. From this point of view the results shown for the two representative TTSs, namely Hcy and β2-m reveal the possible applicability of MAHD for the treatment of CVDs that are motivated by these specific toxins.

Despite these encouraging *in vitro* results we have to mention a current drawback for the case where protein-binding toxins are treated with MAHD. We recall that the results presented in this book were obtained on fHcy, fpC and fβ2-m molecules. In contrast, in blood serum these toxins are not in free form but are primarily bound either with proteins, mainly albumin, or with other candidate molecules. For instance, Hcy readily forms protein-S-S-Hcy conjugates and the dimer homocystine, Hcy-S-S-Hcy, respectively via disulfide bonds. Once these conjugates are formed the chemically active site of the TTSs is already occupied. This will surely prohibit the high affinity of the FN-TBS Cs when the TBS part has almost equivalent chemical reactivity with the protein which is already conjugated with the TTS. Thus, for attaining all the advantages of MAHD more sophisticated TBSs, that should exhibit high affinity for the specific TTSs should be considered in the future. Obviously, the most appropriate TBSs are antibodies.

We hope that the MAHD concept introduced here will motivate Materials-Science and Bioengineering Researchers to investigate new FN-TBS Cs so that very soon our knowledge will be expanded regarding the most appropriate FN-TBS Cs for many TTSs. We also hope that nephrologists will participate in *in vitro* mock-dialysis experiments with donated blood. These experiments are crucial since they will definitely prove the applicability of the proposed concept. Ultimately, *in vivo* applications should be performed where both the efficiency and the biocompatibility of MAHD should be carefully evaluated in animal models.

Hopefully, the future utilization of the MAHD concept in clinical practice, either in the form described in this book or in another more comprehensive approach, could offer to long-term-HD patients all the possible benefits that are discussed here in detail.

References

[1] C.M. Kjellstrand, R.L. Evans, R.J. Peterson, J.R. von Hartitzsch and T.J. Buselmeier "The "unphysiology" of dialysis: A major cause of dialysis side effects?", *Hemodial. Int.* (2004) 8, 24.

[2] F. Locatelli, U. Buoncristiani, B. Canaud, H. Köhler, T. Petitclerc and P. Zucchelli "Dialysis dose and frequency", *Nephrol. Dial. Transplant.* (2005) 20, 285.

[3] U. Buoncristiani, G. Quintiliani, M. Cozzari, L. Giombini and M. Ragaiolo "Daily dialysis: Long-term clinical metabolic results", *Kidney Int.* (1985) 33, S137.

[4] T.A. Depner "Daily hemodialysis efficiency: An analysis of solute kinetics", *Adv. Ren. Replace Ther.* (2001) 8, 227.

[5] R.M. Lindsay and C. Kortas; the Daily/Nocturnal Dialysis Study Group "Hemeral (daily) hemodialysis", *Adv. Ren. Replace Ther.* (2001) 8, 236.

[6] A. Pierratos "Nocturnal home haemodialysis: An update on a 5-year experience", *Nephrol. Dial. Transplant.* (1999) 14, 2835.

[7] A. Pierratos "Daily (quotidian) nocturnal home hemodialysis: Nine years later", *Hemodial Int.* (2004) 8, 45.

[8] A.R. Nissenson, C. Ronco, G. Pergamit, M. Edelstein and R. Watts "The Human Nephron Filter: Toward a Continuously Functioning, Implantable Artificial Nephron System", *Blood Purif.* (2005) 23, 269.

[9] A.R. Nissenson, C. Ronco, G. Pergamit, M. Edelstein and R. Watts "Continuously functioning artificial nephron system: The promise of nanotechnology", *Hemodial. Int.* (2005) 9, 210.

[10] A. Saito "Research into the Development of a Wearable Bioartificial Kidney with a Continuous Hemofilter and a Bioartificial Tubule Device Using Tubular Epithelial Cells", *Artif. Organs* (2004) 28, 58.

[11] P. Aebischer, T.K. Ip, L. Miracoli and P.M. Galletti "Renal epithelial cells grown on semipermeable processor", *Trans. Am. Soc. Artif. Intern. Organs* (1987) 33, 96.

[12] P. Aebischer, T.K. Ip, and P.M. Galletti "The bioartificial kidney: progress toward an ultrafiltration device with renal epithelial cells processing", *Life Support. Sys.* (1987) 5, 159.

[13] H.D. Humes, D.A. Buffington, S.M. MacKay, A.J. Funke and W.F. Weitzel "Replacement of renal function in uremic animals with a tissue-engineering kidney", *Nat. Biotechnol.* (1999) 17, 451.

[14] A. Saito, T. Aung, K. Sekiguchi and Y. Sato "Present Status and Perspective of the Development of a Bioartificial Kidney for Chronic Renal Failure Patients", *Ther. Apher.* (2006) 10, 342.

[15] H.D. Humes, S.M. MacKay, A.J. Funke and D.A. Buffington "Tissue engineering of a bioartificial renal tubule assist device: *In vitro* transport and metabolic characteristics", *Kidney Int.* (1999) 55, 2502.

[16] H.D. Humes, W.H. Fissell and W.F. Weitzel "The bioartificial kidney in the treatment of acute renal failure", *Kidney Int.* (2002) 61, S121.

[17] H.D. Humes, W.F. Weitzel, R.H. Bartlett *et al.* "Initial clinical results of the bioartificial kidney containing human cells in ICU patients with acute renal failure", *Kidney Int.* (2004) 66, 1578.

[18] R. Vanholder and R. De Smet "Pathophysiologic Effects of Uremic Retention Solutes", *J. Am. Soc. Nephrol.* (1999) 10, 1815.

[19] R. Vanholder, A. Argilés, U. Baurmeister *et al.* "Uremic toxicity: Present state of the art", *Int. J. Artif. Organs* (2001) 24, 695.

[20] R. Vanholder, R. De Smet, G. Glorieux *et al.* "Review on uremic toxins: Classification, concentration, and interindividual variability", *Kidney Int.* (2003) 63, 1934.

[21] R. Vanholder, G. Glorieux, R. De Smet and N. Lameire "New insights in uremic toxins", *Kidney Int. Suppl.* (2003) 63, S6.

[22] R. Vanholder, R. De Smet, G. Glorieux and A. Dhondt "Survival of hemodialysis patients and uremic toxin removal", *Artif. Organs* (2003) 27, 218.

[23] H. Refsum, A.D. Smith, P.M. Ueland, E. Nexo, R. Clarke, J. McPartlin, C. Johnston *et al.* "Facts and Recommendations about Total Homocysteine Determinations: An Expert Opinion", *Clin. Chem.* (2004) 50, 3.

[24] D. Shemin, K.L. Lapane, L. Bausserman, E. Kanaan, S. Kahn, L. Dworkin and A.G. Bostom "Plasma total homocysteine and hemodialysis access thrombosis: A prospective study", *J. Am. Soc. Nephrol.* (1999) 10, 1095.

[25] M.E. Suliman, P. Bárány, K. Kalantar-Zadeh, B. Lindholm and P. Stenvinkel "Homocysteine in uraemia - A puzzling and conflicting story", *Nephrol. Dial. Transpl.* (2005) 20, 16.

[26] F. Pizzolo, S. Friso, O. Olivieri, N. Martinelli, C. Bozzini, P. Guarini, E. Trabetti, G. Faccini, R. Corrocher and D. Girelli "Homocysteine, traditional risk factors and impaired renal function in coronary artery disease", *Eur. J. Clin. Invest.* (2006) 36, 698.

[27] M. Suliman, P. Stenvinkel, A.R. Qureshi, K. Kalantar-Zadeh, P. Bárány, O. Heimbürger, E.F. Vonesh and B. Lindholm "The reverse epidemiology of plasma total homocysteine as a mortality risk factor is related to the impact of wasting and inflammation", *Nephrol. Dial. Transpl.* (2007) 22, 209.

[28] F. Gejyo, T. Yamada, S. Odani *et al.* "A new form of amyloid protein associated with chronic hemodialysis was identified as β2-microglobulin", *Biochem. Biophys. Res. Commun.* (1985) 129, 701.

[29] P.D. Gorevic, T.T. Casey, W.J. Stone, C.R. Diraimondo, F.C. Prelli and B. Frangione "Beta−2 microglobulin is an amyloidogenic protein in man", *J. Clin. Invest.* (1985) 76, 2425.

[30] T.B. Drüeke "β2-Microglobulin and amyloidosis", *Nephrol. Dial. Transpl. Suppl. 1* (2000) 15, 17.

[31] C. Ronco and A.R. Nissenson "Does Nanotechnology Apply to Dialysis?", *Blood Purif.* (2001) 19, 347.

[32] H.D. Humes, W.H. Fissell and K. Tiranathanagul "The future of hemodialysis membranes", *Kidney Int.* (2006) 69, 1115.

[33] W.H. Fissell, H.D. Humes, A.J. Fleischman and S. Roy "Dialysis and Nanotechnology: Now, 10 Years, or Never?", *Blood Purif.* (2007) 25, 12.

[34] D. Stamopoulos, D. Benaki, P. Bouziotis and P.N. Zirogiannis "In vitro utilization of ferromagnetic nanoparticles in hemodialysis therapy", *Nanotechnology* (2007) 18, 495102.

[35] D. Stamopoulos "Magnetic Nanoparticles Utilized in Hemodialysis for the Treatment of Hyperhomocysteinemia: The New Challenge of Nanobiotechnology", *Curr. Nanosci.* (2008) 4, 301.

[36] D. Stamopoulos, P. Bouziotis, D. Benaki, P.N. Zirogiannis, K. Kotsovassilis, V. Belessi, V. Dalamagas and K. Papadopoulos "Magnetically Assisted Haemodialysis for the Prevention of Dialysis-Related Amyloidosis", submitted for publication.

[37] D. Stamopoulos, P. Bouziotis, D. Benaki, C. Kotsovassilis and P.N. Zirogiannis "Utilization of nanobiotechnology in haemodialysis: mock-dialysis experiments on homocysteine", *Nephrol. Dial. Transpl.* (2007) doi: 10.1093/ndt/gfn189.

[38] D. Stamopoulos, M. Pissas, V. Karanasos, D. Niarchos and I. Panagiotopoulos "Influence of randomly distributed magnetic nanoparticles on surface superconductivity in Nb films", *Phys. Rev. B* (2004) 70, 054512.

[39] D. Stamopoulos and E. Manios "Superconducting-Ferromagnetic Hybrid Structures and their Possible Applications" Chapter 4 in book "Superconductivity, Magnetism and Magnets", NOVA Science Publisher, New York (2006).

[40] A.B. Bourlinos, A. Bakandritsos, V. Georgakilas, V. Tzitzios and D. Petridis "Facile synthesis of capped γ-Fe_2O_3 and Fe_3O_4 nanoparticles", *J. Mater. Sci.* (2006) 41, 5250.

[41] D. Stamopoulos, M. Pissas and E. Manios "Ferromagnetic-superconducting hybrid films and their possible applications: A direct study in a model combinatorial film", *Phys. Rev. B* (2005) 71, 014522.

[42] D. Stamopoulos, E. Manios, M. Pissas and D. Niarchos "Pronounced T_c enhancement and magnetic memory effects in hybrid films", *Supercond. Sci. Tech.* (2004) 17, L51-L54.

[43] N. Noginova, T. Weaver, M. King, A.B. Bourlinos, E.P. Giannelis and V.A. Atsarkin "NMR and spin relaxation in systems with magnetic nanoparticles", *J. Phys.: Condens. Mat.* (2007) 19, 076210.

[44] D. Stamopoulos, D. Benaki and P. Bouziotis "Physical properties of magnetic nanoparticles-BSA conjugates: from drug delivery to contrast agents", submitted for publication.

[45] Y.-W. Jun, Y.-M. Huh, J.-S. Choi *et al.* "Nanoscale Size Effect of Magnetic Nanocrystals and Their Utilization for Cancer Diagnosis via Magnetic Resonance Imaging", *J. Am. Chem. Soc.* (2005) 127, 5732.

[46] Y.-M. Huh, Y.-W. Jun, H.-T. Song *et al.* "In vivo magnetic resonance detection of cancer by using multifunctional magnetic nanocrystals", *J. Am. Chem. Soc.* (2005) 127, 12387.

[47] U.O. Hafeli, S.M. Sweeney, B.A. Beresford, J.L. Humm and R.M. Macklis "Effective targeting of magnetic radioactive ^{90}Y-microspheres to tumor cells by an externally applied magnetic field. Preliminary *in vitro* and *in vivo* results", *Nucl. Med. Biol.* (1995) 22, 147.

[48] J. Chen, H. Wu, D. Han and C. Xie "Using anti-VEGF McAb and magnetic nanoparticles as double-targeting vector for the radioimmunotherapy of liver cancer", *Cancer Lett.* (2006) 231, 169.

[49] Y.W. Cho, S.A. Park, T.H. Han *et al.* "*In vivo* tumor targeting and radionuclide imaging with self-assembled nanoparticles: Mechanisms, key factors, and their implications", *Biomaterials* (2007) 28, 1236.

[50] S. Mornet, S. Vasseur, F. Grasset and E. Duguet "Magnetic nanoparticle design for medical diagnosis and therapy", *J. Mater. Chem.* (2004) 14, 2161.

[51] C.C. Berry and A.S.G. Curtis "Functionalization of magnetic nanoparticles for applications in biomedicine", *J. Phys. D: Appl. Phys.* (2003) 36, R198.

[52] P. Tartaj, M.P. Morales, S. Veintemillas-Verdaguer and T. González-Carreño "The preparation of magnetic nanoparticles for applications in biomedicine", *J. Phys. D: Appl. Phys.* (2003) 36, R182.

[53] A.K. Gupta and M. Gupta "Synthesis and surface engineering of iron oxide nanoparticles for biomedical applications", *Biomaterials* (2005) 26, 3995.

[54] M. Shinkai "Functional magnetic particles for medical application", *J. Biosci. Bioeng.* (2002) 94, 606.

[55] H.E. Horng, S.Y. Yang, C.Y. Hong, C.M. Liu, P.S. Tsai, H.C. Yang and C. C. Wu "Biofunctionalized magnetic nanoparticles for high-sensitivity immunomagnetic detection of human C-reactive protein", *Appl. Phys. Lett.* (2006) 88, 252506.

[56] C.Y. Hong, W.S. Chen, Z.F. Jian, S.Y. Yang, H.E. Horng, L.C. Yang and H.C. Yang "Wash-free immunomagnetic detection for serum through magnetic susceptibility reduction", *Appl. Phys. Lett.* (2007) 90, 074105.

[57] C.C. Wu, B.F. Hong, B.H. Wu *et al.* "Animal magnetocardiography using superconducting quantum interference device gradiometers assisted with magnetic nanoparticle injection: A sensitive method for early detecting electromagnetic changes induced by hypercholesterolemia", *Appl. Phys. Lett.* (2007) 90, 054111.

[58] B.G. Danielson "Structure, Chemistry, and Pharmacokinetics of Intravenous Iron Agents", *J. Am. Soc. Nephrol.* (2004) 15, S93.

[59] D. Choundhury and Z. Ahmed "Drug-associated renal dysfunction and injury", *Nat. Clin. Pract. Nephrol.* (2006) 2, 80.

[60] L.J. McWilliam "Drug-induced renal disease", *Curr. Diagn. Pathol.* (2007) 13, 25.

[61] L. Wang, Z. Yang, J. Gao, K. Xu, H. Gu, B. Zhang, X. Zhang and B. Xu "A biocompatible method of decorporation: Bisphosphonate-modified magnetite nanoparticles to remove uranyl ions from blood", *J. Am. Chem. Soc.* (2006) 128, 13358.

[62] A.S. Levey, J. Coresh, E. Balk, A.T. Kausz, A. Levin, M.W. Steffes, R.J. Hogg, R.D. Perrone, J. Lau and G. Eknoyan "National Kidney Foundation Practice Guidelines for Chronic Kidney Disease: Evaluation, Classification, and Stratification", *Ann. Intern. Med.* (2003) 139, 137.

[63] A.S. Levey, J. Coresh, T. Greene, L.A. Stevens, Y. Zhang, S. Hendriksen, J.W. Kusek and F. Van Lente "Using Standardized Serum Creatinine Values in the Modification of Diet in Renal Disease Study Equation for Estimating Glomerular Filtration Rate", *Ann. Intern. Med.* (2006) 145, 247.

[64] NKF-DOQI, National Kidney Foundation, *Am. J. Kidney Dis.* (1997) 30 S67; NKF-K/DOQI, Update 2000, *Am. J. Kidney Dis.* (2001) 37, S7.

[65] A.S. Levey, J.P. Bosch, J.B. Lewis, T. Greene, N. Rogers and D. Roth "A more accurate method to estimate glomerular filtration rate from serum creatinine: A new prediction equation", *Ann. Intern. Med.* (1999) 130, 461.

[66] A.S. Levey, T. Greene, G.J. Beck, A.W. Caggiula, J.W. Kusek, L.G. Hunsicker and S. Klahr "Dietary protein restriction and the progression of chronic renal disease: What have all of the results of the MDRD study shown?", *J. Am. Soc. Nephrol.* (1999) 10, 2426.

[67] A.S. Levey, T. Greene, J.W. Kusek and G. Beck "A simplified equation to predict glomerular filtration rate from serum creatinine" (Abstract), *J. Am. Soc. Nephrol.* (2000) 11, A828.

[68] V. Bonomini, C. Feletti, M.P. Scolari and S. Stefoni "Benefits of early initiation of dialysis", *Kidney Int. Suppl.* (1985) 17, S57.

[69] J. Tattersall, R. Greenwood and K. Farrington "Urea kinetics and when to commence dialysis", *Am. J. Nephrol.* (1995) 15, 283.

[70] D.N. Churchill, K.E. Thorpe, E.F. Vonesh and R.R. Keshaviah "Lower probability of patient survival and continuous peritoneal dialysis in the United States compared with Canada", *J. Am. Soc. Nephrol.* (1997) 8, 965.

[71] D.N. Churchill "An evidence-based approach to earlier initiation of dialysis", *Am. J. Kidney Dis.* (1997) 30, 899.

[72] G.T. Obrador and B.J.G. Pereira "Early referral to the nephrologist and timely initiation of renal replacement therapy: A paradigm shift in the management of patients with chronic renal failure", *Am. J. Kidney Dis.* (1998) 31, 398.

[73] J.P. Traynor, K. Simpson, C.C. Geddes, C.J. Deighan and J.G. Fox "Early initiation of dialysis fails to prolong survival in patients with end-stage renal failure", *J. Am. Soc. Nephrol.* (2002) 13, 2125.

[74] J.C. Korevaar, M.A. Jansen, F.W. Dekker, K.J. Jager, E.W. Boeschoten, R.T. Krediet and P.M. Bossuyt "When to initiate dialysis: Effect of proposed US guidelines on survival", *Lancet* (2001) 358, 1046.

[75] J.C. Fink, R.A. Burdick, S.J. Kurth, S.A. Blahut, N.C. Armistead, M.S. Turner, L.M. Shickle and P.D. Light "Significance of serum creatinine values in new end-stage renal disease patients", *Am. J. Kidney Dis.* (1999) 34, 694.

[76] S. Beddhu, M.H. Samore, M.S. Roberts, G.J. Stoddard, N. Ramkumar, L.M. Pappas and A.K. Cheung "Impact of timing of initiation of dialysis on mortality", *J. Am. Soc. Nephrol.* (2003) 14, 2305.

[77] J.K. Leypoldt, A.K. Cheung, L.Y. Agodoa, J.T. Daugirdas, T. Greene, P.R. Keshaviah and G.J. Beck "Hemodialyzer mass transfer-area coefficients for urea increase at high dialysate flow rates", *Kidney Int.* (1997) 51, 2013.

[78] T. Greene, G.J. Beck, J.J. Gassman, F.A. Gotch, J.W. Kusek, A.S. Levey, N.W. Levin, G. Schulman and G. Eknoyan "Design and statistical issues of The Hemodialysis (HEMO) Study", *Control Clin. Trials* (2000) 21, 502.

[79] G. Eknoyan, G.J. Beck, A.K. Cheung *et al.* "Effect of dialysis dose and membrane flux in maintenance hemodialysis", *N. Engl. J. Med.* (2002) 347, 2010.

[80] B.H. Scridner and D.G. Oreopoulos "The hemodialysis product (HDP): A better index of dialysis adequacy than Kt/V", *Dialysis Transplant.* (2002) 31, 13.

[81] W.J. Johnson, W.W. Hagge, R.D. Wagoner, R.P. Dinapoli and J.W. Rosevear "Effects of urea loading in patients with far advanced renal failure", *Mayo Clin. Proc.* (1972) 47, 21.

[82] R.A. Ward and C. Ronco "Dialyzer and Machine Technologies: Application of Recent Advances to Clinical Practice", *Blood Purificat.* (2006) 24, 6.

[83] A.K. Cheung, N.W. Levin, T. Greene *et al.* "Effects of High-Flux Hemodialysis on Clinical Outcomes: Results of the HEMO Study", *J. Am. Soc. Nephrol.* (2003) 14, 3251.

[84] R. Vanholder, R. De Smet, M.A. Waterloos, N. Van Landschoot, P. Vogeleere, E. Hoste and S. Ringoir "Mechanisms of uremic inhibition of phagocyte reactive species production: Characterization of the role of *p*-cresol", *Kidney Int.* (1995) 47, 510.

[85] R. De Smet, J. Van Kaer, B. Van Vlem, A. De Cubber, P. Brunet, N. Lameire and R. Vanholder "Toxicity of Free *p*-Cresol: A Prospective and Cross-Sectional Analysis", *Clin. Chem.* (2003) 49, 470.

[86] T. Bardin, J. Zingraff, D. Kuntz and T. Drueke "Dialysis - Related amyloidosis", *J. Clin. Invest.* (1986) 1, 151.

[87] C. van Ypersele de Strihou, B. Honhon, J.M. Vandenbroucke, J.P. Huaux, H. No¨el and B. Maldague "Dialysis amyloidosis", *Adv. Nephrol.* (1988) 17, 401.

[88] T. Miyata, O. Oda, R. Inagi, Y. Iida, N. Araki, N. Yamada, S. Horiuchi, N. Taniguchi, K. Maeda and T. Kinoshita "β2-Microglobulin modified with advanced glycation end products is a major component of hemodialysis-associated amyloidosis", *J. Clin. Invest.* (1993) 92, 1243.

[89] T. Miyata, Y. Iida, Y. Ueda, T. Shinzato, H. Seo, V.M. Monnier, K. Maeda and Y. Wada "Monocyte/macrophage response to β2-microglobulin modified with advanced glycation end products", *Kidney Int.* (1996) 49, 538.

[90] T.B. Drüeke "Dialysis-related amyloidosis", *Nephrol. Dial. Transpl.* (1998) 13, 58.

[91] A. Benkert, F. Scheller, W. Schossler, C. Hentschel, B. Micheel, O. Behrsing, G. Scharte, W. Stocklein and A. Warsinke "Development of a creatinine ELISA and an amperometric antibody-based creatinine sensor with a detection limit in the nanomolar range", *Anal. Chem.* (2000) 72, 916.

[92] See www.abcam.com

[93] B. Canaud, L. Chenine, H. Leray-Moragués, H. Wiesen and C. Tetta "Residual renal function and dialysis modality: Is it really beneficial to preserve residual renal function in dialysis patients?", *Nephrology* (2006) 11, 292.

[94] A.M. Hung, B.S. Young and G.M. Chertow "The Decline in Residual Renal Function in Hemodialysis Is Slow and Age Dependent", *Hemodial. Int.* (2003) 7, 17.

[95] S.M. Chandna and K. Farrington "Residual renal function: Considerations on its importance and preservation in dialysis patients", *Semin. Dial.* (2004) 17, 196.

[96] B. Charra "'Dry weight' in dialysis: the history of a concept", *Nephrol. Dial. Transpl.* (1998) 13, 1882.

[97] B.G. Stegmayr "Ultrafiltration and Dry Weight-What Are the Cardiovascular Effects?", *Artif. Organs* (2003) 27, 227.

[98] E.F. Molaison and M.K. Yadrick "Stages of change and fluid intake in dialysis patients", *Patient Educ. Couns.* (2003) 49, 5.

[99] J. Scheuer and S.W. Stezoski "The effect of uraemic compounds on cardiac function and metabolism", *J. Mol. Cell. Cardiol.* (1973) 5, 287.

[100] W. Norde and C.E. Giacomelli "BSA structural changes during homomolecular exchange between the absorbed and the dissolved states", *J. Biotechnol.* (2000) 79, 259.

[101] C.E. Giacomelli and W. Norde "The Adsorption-Desorption Cycle. Reversibility of the BSA-Silica System", *J. Colloid. Interface Sci.* (2001) 233, 233.

[102] N. Shamim, L. Hong, K. Hidajat and M.S. Uddin "Thermosensitive-polymer-coated magnetic nanoparticles: Adsorption and desorption of Bovine Serum Albumin", *J. Colloid. Interface Sci.* (2006) 304, 1.

[103] M. Mikhaylova, D.K. Kim, C.C. Berry, A. Zagorodni, M. Toprak, A.S.G. Curtis and M. Muhammed "BSA Immobilization on Amine-Functionalized Superparamagnetic Iron Oxide Nanoparticles", *Chem. Mater.* (2004) 16, 2344.

[104] E.P. Furlani and K.C. Ng "Analytical model of magnetic nanoparticle transport and capture in the microvasculature", *Phys. Rev. E* (2006) 73, 061919.

[105] H.S. Choi, W. Liu, P. Misra, E. Tanaka, J.P. Zimmer, B. I. Ipe, M.G. Bawendi and J.V. Frangioni "Renal clearance of quantum dots", *Nat. Biotechnol.* (2007) 25, 1165.

[106] M. Arruedo, R. Fernández-Pacheco, M. Ricardo Ibarra and J. Santamaria "Magnetic nanoparticles for drug delivery", *Nano Today* (2007) 2, 22.

[107] R.S. Tu and V. Breedveld "Microrheological detection of protein unfolding" *Phys. Rev. E* (2005) 72, 041914.

[108] M.R. Wattenbarger, V.A. Bloomfield, Z. Bu and P.S. Russo "Tracer diffusion of proteins in DNA solutions", *Macromolecules* (1992) 25, 5263.

[109] See chapter 5 in J.D. Jackson "Classical Electrodynamics", 3rd Edition, John Wiley and Sons, New York (2001).

[110] S.R. Lentz "Mechanisms of thrombosis in hyperhomocysteinemia", *Curr. Opin. Hematol.* (1998) 5, 343.

[111] S.R. Lentz "Mechanisms of homocysteine-induced atherothrombosis", *J. Thromb. Haemost.* (2005) 3, 1646.

[112] W.G. Haynes "Hyperhomocysteinemia, vascular function and atherosclerosis: Effects of vitamins", *Cardiovasc. Drugs Ther.* (2002) 16, 391.

[113] H. Refsum, P.M. Ueland, O. Nygård and S.E. Vollset "Homocysteine and cardiovascular disease", *Annu. Rev. Med.* (1998) 49, 31.

[114] O. Nygård, S.E. Vollset, H. Refsum, L. Brattström and P.M. Ueland "Total homocysteine and cardiovascular disease", *J. Intern. Med.* (1999) 246, 425.

[115] J.W. Eikelboom, E. Lonn, Jr. J. Genest, G. Hankey and S. Yusuf "Homocyst(e)ine and cardiovascular disease: A critical review of the epidemiologic evidence", *Ann. Intern. Med.* (1999) 131, 363.

[116] D.W. Jacobsen "Homocysteine and vitamins in cardiovascular disease", *Clin. Chem.* (1998) 44, 1833.

[117] A.G. Bostom, D. Shemin, P. Verhoef *et al.* "Elevated plasma homocysteine levels and cardiovascular disease outcomes in maintenance dialysis patients. A prospective study", *Arterioscler. Thromb. Vasc. Biol.* (1997) 17, 2554.

[118] F. Mallamaci, C. Zoccali, G. Triperi *et al.* "Hyperhomocysteinemia predicts cardiovascular outcomes in hemodialysis patients", *Kidney Int.* (2002) 61, 609.

[119] E. Nurk, H. Refsum, G.S. Tell, K. Engedal, S.E. Vollset, P.M. Ueland, H.A. Nygaard and A.D. Smith "Plasma total homocysteine and memory in the elderly: The Hordaland homocysteine study", *Ann. Neurol.* (2005) 58, 847.

[120] A. McCaddon, G. Davies, P. Hudson, S. Tandy and H. Cattell "Total serum homocysteine in senile dementia of Alzheimer type", *Int. J. Geriatr. Psych.* (1998) 13, 235.

[121] S. Seshadri "Elevated plasma homocysteine levels: Risk factor or risk marker for the development of dementia and Alzheimer's disease?", *J. Alz. Dis.* (2006) 9, 393.

[122] C. van Guldener "Why is homocysteine elevated in renal failure and what can be expected from homocysteine-lowering?", *Nephrol. Dial. Transpl.* (2006) 21, 1161.

[123] C. van Guldener, M.J. Janssen, J. Lambert *et al.* "No change in impaired endothelial function after long-term folic acid therapy of hyperhomocysteinaemia in hemodialysis patients", *Nephrol. Dial. Transpl.* (1998) 13, 106.

[124] S. Doshi, I. McDowell, S. Moat, M. Lewis and J. Goodfellow "Folate improves endothelial function in patients with coronary heart disease", *Clin. Chem. Lab. Med.* (2003) 41, 1505.

[125] J.P. Glusker "Structural aspects of metal liganding to functional groups in proteins", *Adv. Prot. Chem.* (1991) 42, 1.

[126] J.B. Howard and D.C. Rees "Perspectives on non-heme iron protein chemistry", *Adv. Prot. Chem.* (1991) 42, 199.

[127] D. Carter and J. Ho "Serum Albumin", *Adv. Prot. Chem.* (1994) 45, 153.

[128] T. Peters Jr. "All about Albumin: Biochemistry, Genetics, and Medical Applications", Academic Press, San Diego, CA (1996).

[129] F.X. Zhang, L. Han, L.B. Israel, J.G. Daras, M.M. Maye, N.K. Ly and C.-J. Zhong "Colorimetric detection of thiol-containing amino acids using gold nanoparticles", *Analyst* (2002) 127, 462.

[130] A. Abbaspour and R. Mirzajami "Indirect Simultaneous Kinetic Determination of L-Cysteine and Homocysteine by ANNs", *Anal. Lett.* (2006) 39, 791.

[131] I.-I.S. Lim, S. Lim, W. Ip, E. Crew, P.N. Njoki, D. Mott, C.-J. Zhong, Y. Pan and S. Zhou "Homocysteine-mediated reactivity and assembly of gold nanoparticles", *Langmuir* (2007) 23, 826.

[132] X. He and D.C. Carter "Atomic structure and chemistry of human serum albumin", *Nature* (1992) 358, 209.

[133] U. Kragh-Hansen, V.T.G. Chuang and M. Otagiri "Practical Aspects of the Ligand-Binding and Enzymatic Properties of Human Serum Albumin", *Biol. Pharm. Bull.* (2002) 25, 695.

[134] S. Sengupta, H. Chen, T. Togawa, P.M. DiBello, A.K. Majors, B. Büdy, M.E. Ketterer and D.W. Jacobsen "Albumin Thiolate Anion Is an Intermediate in the Formation of Albumin-S-S-Homocysteine", *J. Biol. Chem.* (2001) 276, 30111.

[135] M.T. Shipchandler and E.G. Moore "Rapid, Fully Automated Measurements of Plasma Homocyst(e)ine with the Abbott IMx® Analyzer", *Clin. Chem.* (1995) 41, 991.

[136] P. Pernet, E. Lasnier and M. Vaubourdolle "Evaluation of the AxSYM Homocysteine Assay and Comparison with the IMx Homocysteine Assay", *Clin. Chem.* (2000) 46, 1440.

[137] NKF-K/DOQI Clinical Practice Guidelines for the Treatment of Anemia of Chronic Renal Failure. New York, National Kidney Foundation, 2000.

[138] T. Niwa "Phenol and p-cresol accumulated in uremic serum measured by HPLC with fluorescence detection", *Clin. Chem.* (1993) 39, 108.

[139] G. Lesaffer, R.D. Smet, N. Lameire *et al.* "Intradialytic removal of protein-bound uraemic toxins: role of solute characteristics and of dialyser membrane", *Nephrol. Dial. Transpl.* (2000) 15, 50.

[140] J. Stange, W. Ramlow, S. Mitzner, R. Schmidt and H. Klinkmann "Dialysis against a recycled albumin solution enables the removal of albumin-bound toxins", *Artif. Organs* (1993) 17, 809.

[141] T. Abe, T. Abe, S. Ageta, T. Kakuta, N. Suzuki, H. Hirata, M. Shouno, H. Saio and T. Akizawa "A New Method for Removal of Albumin-Binding Uremic Toxins: Efficiency of an Albumin-Dialysate", *Ther. Apher.* (2001) 5, 58.

[142] J.W. Becker and G.N. Reeke, Jr. "Three-dimensional structure of β_2-microglobulin", *Proc. Natl. Acad. Sci. USA* (1985) 82, 4225.

[143] C.H. Trinh, D.P. Smith, A.P. Kalverda, S.E.V. Phillips and S.E. Radford "Crystal structure of monomeric human $\beta - 2$-microglobulin reveals clues to its amyloidogenic properties", *Proc. Natl. Acad. Sci. USA* (2002) 99, 9771.

[144] B. Ma and R. Nussinov "Molecular dynamics simulations of the unfolding of β_2-microglobulin and its variants", *Protein Eng.* (2003) 16, 561.

[145] F. Gejyo, S. Odani and T. Yamada "β2-microglobulin: A new form of amyloid protein associated with chronic hemodialysis", *Kidney Int.* (1986) 30, 385.

[146] P.D. Gorevic, T.T. Casey, W.J. Stone, C.R. Diraimondo, F.C. Prelli, B. Frangione "Beta-2 microglobulin is an amyloidogenic protein in man", *J Clin. Inv.* (1985) 76, 2425.

[147] A. Saito and F. Gejyo "Current Clinical Aspects of Dialysis-Related Amyloidosis in Chronic Dialysis Patients", *Ther. Apher.* (2006) 10, 316.

[148] de Strihou C. van Ypersele, M. Jadoul, J. Malghem, B. Maldague, J. Jamart "Effect of dialysis membrane and patient's age on signs of dialysis-related amyloidosis. The Working Party on Dialysis Amyloidosis", *Kidney Int.* (1991) 39, 1012.

[149] I. Aoike, F. Gejyo and M. Arakawa "Learning from the Japanese Registry: how will we prevent long-term complications? Niigata Research Programme for beta2-M Removal Membrane", *Nephrol. Dial. Transplant.* (1995) 10, 7.

[150] Y. Koda, S. Nishi, S. Miyazaki, et al. "Switch from conventional to high-flux membrane reduces the risk of carpal tunnel syndrome and mortality of hemodialysis patients", *Kidney Int.* (1997) 52, 1096.

[151] A.C. Fry, D.K. Singh, S.M. Chandna and K. Farrington "Relative Importance of Residual Renal Function and Convection in Determining Bate-2-Microglobulin Levels in High-Flux Haemodialysis and On-Line Haemodiafiltration", *Blood Purif* (2007) 25, 295.

[152] A. Saito, J.J. Kazama, N. Iino et al. "Bioengineered implantation of megalin-expressing cells: a potential intracorporeal therapeutic model for uremic toxin protein clearance in renal failure.", *J Am. Soc. Nephrol.* (2003) 14, 2025.

[153] L. Thomas "Immunological Technics" In: L. Thomas "Clinical laboratory diagnostics. Use and assessment of clinical laboratory results" 1st edition. TH-Books, Frankfurt/Main, Germany, 1198.

Index

E

F

G

H

I

O

P

Q

R

S

T

U

V

W

X